Survival Collection:
First Aid Medications, Hacks, Tips and Tools to Keep You Safe

Table of content

Survival Communication

Introduction

Survival communication during tough situations is really necessary as without it, you will not be able to get out of tensed situation. Mobile phone communications have a ton of vulnerabilities like being subject to mobile locales which can be influenced in catastrophes like surges and earth tremors, low battery life, and so on, which makes it a poor decision for communication for long-term crises. As specified before, substantial winds and flooding can upset mobile towers and links bringing on the loss of sign like what happened during Hurricane Sandy and many other natural calamities as well. Mobile locales or towers works on AC control only and this can be a major issue when the fundamental force source is upset which is generally the case during trips.

Most mobile towers use generators for reinforcement power supply however generators are the fleeting plan as they require fuel that must be renewed again and again. Mobile phone communication relies on back pull frameworks that are not generally strong since they are wired which can, in any case, be influenced by surges and earth quacks. Mobile phones have a short battery life which would keep going for a day or three. This can be a major issue for long term debacles or emergency since you won't have the capacity to make use of your PDA unless you have a local energy source to back it up.

Mobile phones oblige satellites to build up a steady flag for communication. Shockingly satellites are defenseless against physical assaults, programs, and sunlight based tempests. Whenever force and business lines are down, the best way to have the capacity to interface with the outside world is by utilizing radios as emergency communication gear. Since they don't rely on upon AC force, satellites, or business lines, so they require alternatives to set up a sign for communication.

Chapter 1 – Communication for survival in intense situation

If you get yourself stuck in any disaster and there is no way out then, you must be thinking the way by which you can communicate with your family. Definitely, when you are facing a kind of calamity and there is no one to help you out then you will require something to communicate to your family for sure. In that situation, you cannot just rely on the use of mobile phones. This is because there may be a chance that your mobile battery goes down or may be the place where you reside does not have mobile towers to transmit signals. So, you must look for some kind of alternatives to communicate with your friends and family.

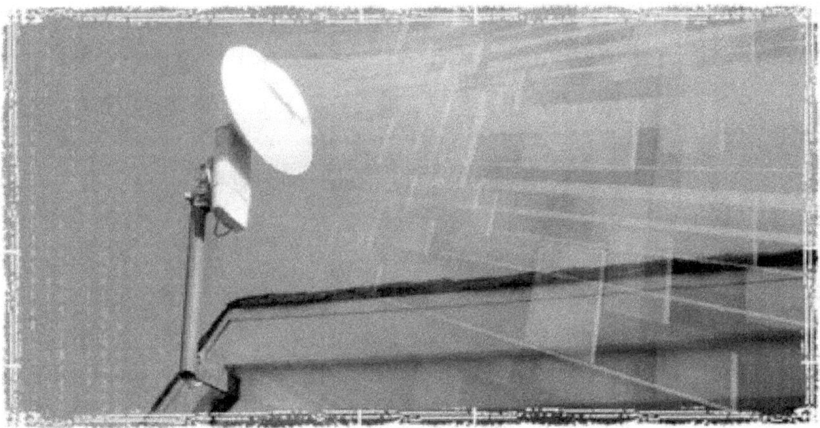

Here, I am going to discuss several ways by which you can communicate with your loved ones and can call them to take you out of that calamity you are facing. Crises which is short-term have demonstrated the impediments of making use of phones to have proper communication with each other. Regardless of the possibility that the towers are operational, they can't deal with the additional movement of so many individuals, who attempt to take a few things to get back to some composure of friends and family or help.

How to communicate during a crisis?

During so many occasions which have occurred recently, the services of mobile phones cannot be taken as the most important option for quite a long time. The framework turned out to be genuinely over-burdened on 9/11 so calls failed to be made. 70% of the towers went down during the flood Katrina and were down for a considerable length of time, and most territories haven't been satisfactorily enhanced throughout the Unites States.

These won't be detached occasions. Try not to believe that since you live in a substantial metropolitan region, you will find yourself more secure. Take a look at a portion of the things that continued during Hurricane Sandy in New York. This will demonstrate that the legislature has a lot of things to manage by simply attempting to recover your phone service up so, despite the fact that that was an entirely transient occasion, it brought on a lot of issues.

- Phone correspondence has a great deal of susceptibilities that mark it a pitiable answer for far-reaching or long-lasting crises.

- Substantial airstreams or water overflowing can upset the links between towers, for example, for the duration of Hurricane Sandy.

Mobile towers have need of AC energy to work so in case they don't have a programmed reinforcement framework, they stop. Remember that a wide range of towers are simply celebrated radio wires on the highest points of structures or foothills and reinforcement force, for example, a backup generator is a fleeting plan. Generators entail fuel and that oil must be recharged frequently. In many circumstances, the main reinforcement power which is accessible is a store of batteries that twitch charging as soon as the primary force framework stops.

Back term frameworks that are basically the framework that interfaces or permits flood from external frameworks to the center, regularly include different transporters, aren't generally strong. A great deal of this framework is supported however has been extended to the microwave and different frameworks as well.

Most mobile phones will just remain charged for a couple of days. In case you don't have the local energy to retain it high, when the framework comes move down, you won't have the capacity to converse with it. Mobile phones have need of outposts, that are defenseless against programs, physical assault, or sun oriented tempests. They'll be truly pointless if the countrywide framework goes down because of a digital assault, CME or EMP, that is significantly more probable than you may suspect.

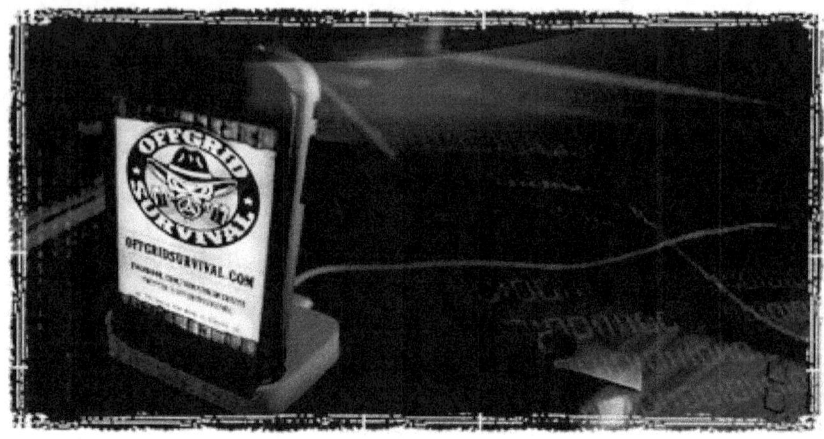

One cool thought that is turning on view is the goTenna mobile phone radio wire framework. Your mobile phone interfaces with it by means of Bluetooth and an application, and the sign is sent and got through a scrambled radio sign. It won't have the capacity to reach to the opposite side of a city however you ought to have the capacity to find your family in case they're in the territory and perhaps speak with others in case they have the framework.

Chapter 2 – How to communicate during worse situations?

There can be so many options that should be taken into consideration by you if you are looking for survival communication. Here are some of the devices which will help you in communication without trouble.

CB radio

Many people developed up viewing the Bear and BJ and they saw every one of the haulers having conversation over the air with one another. CB radio is certainly more accessible during an emergency but they have a lot of restrictions.

According to some, not many individuals are on CB. You may have the capacity to discover somebody in a wagon however even that is harder to discover. The issue isn't only the absence of individuals who utilize it, it's the absence of individuals in your reach that make use of it.

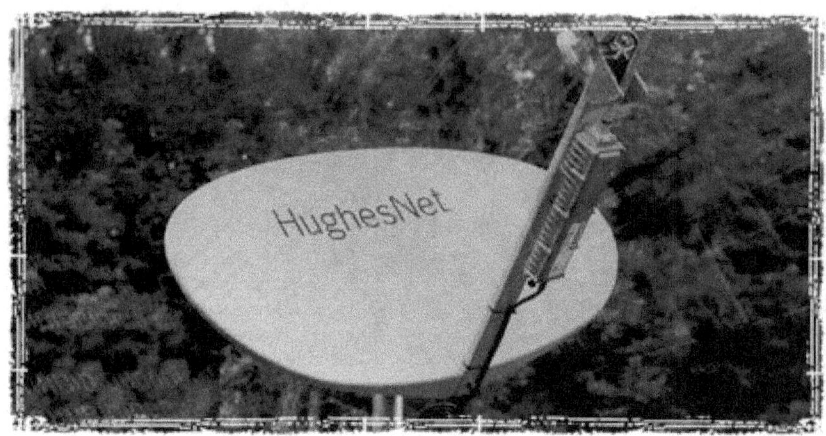

Amongst the enormous reasons your extent is extremely restricted with CB versus different frameworks is that they're constrained to input of 5 watts which is around output of 4 watt. It might be only some dubious thought but additional power results in more unglued. At the regularities that CB transistors utilizes, you can just hope to get somewhere sandwiched between 1 and 10 loads or miles or something like that, contingent upon the landscape. There can be a billion people in the Unites States with their CB's all on the similar network in the meantime, but in case they do not inside reach, you won't talk.

You may imagine that you can simply scribbler into your veal radio and thrust out extra control, however the FCC follows individuals who try to do that in only a couple of cases. Clearly with SHTF, you're not going to truly think around that however rather recall that addition with more energy to transmit. Also, to get more remote doesn't do whatever to benefit you listens to the former person with an ordinary CB transmitter.

Should you opt for satellite phone for an emergency?

In many emergency circumstances, the satellite phones are quite great. The primary issue with them, however, is an expense. They're really very costly. Not just do you need to spend for the phone, you need to recompense for package and minutes. In case you're stranded at some place, it may be justified regardless of the expense.

They don't generally work, however. You should have one with you at all times, and it will come in a hell of convenience. They don't care for wildernesses however because of the trees obstructing the satellites and in opposition to what each cracking film appears, they don't work inside a boat like they continued appearing in World War Z.

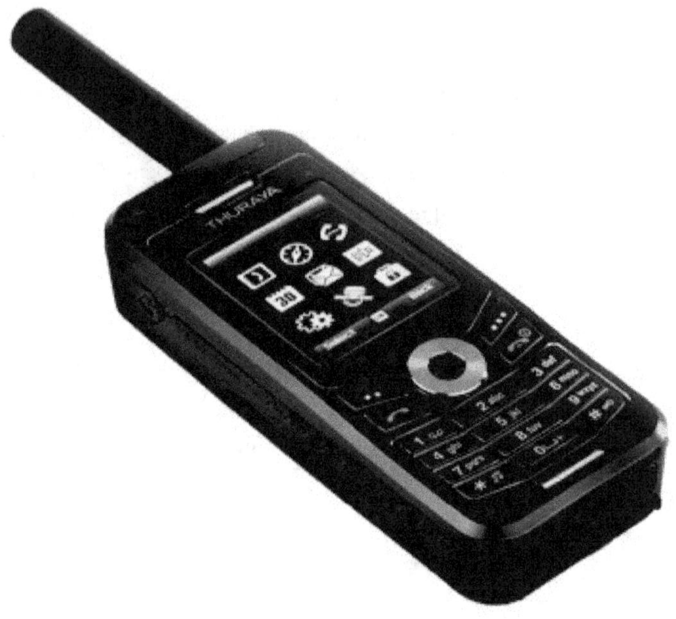

The genuine issue is that it's very improbable that you'd need it in an ordinary family unit so they're only useful for crises and most likely they are not worth the expense. Another enormous issue is that simply like mobile phones, they be determined by on the outposts to have a great capacity so if the outposts quit functioning, the satellite phones will also do the same. Clearly. Sunlight based tempests and CMEs have reserved out satellites previously. They will do it once more.

GMRS radios

For nearby correspondence, MURS radios and GMRS and FRS are truly great. They don't require an FCC permit for MURS and FRS, they're tranquil to operate and simple to be understood. They've basically substituted CB radios for a considerable measure of families. In that capacity, despite the fact that they're a change, they have a ton of the same restriction on force and range.

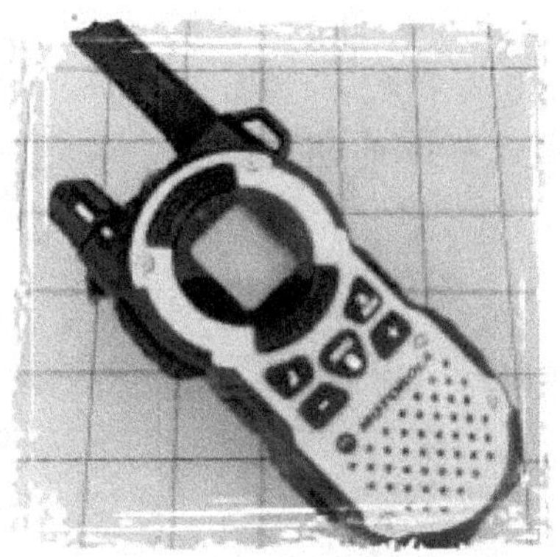

In case you have a genuine GMRS radio, you might possess the capacity to take benefit of a repeater that will extend your reach to conceivably several miles. But, the repeater clearly must run, and you must be within the scope for your radio's repeater to knockout it. GMRS transistors are likewise permitted to work at a higher force than a considerable measure of different radios. You likewise require a permit to make use of GMRS frequencies. Fundamentally, in case you're thinking about one of these radio frameworks to be used in an emergency, you should opt for a genuine GMRS transistor and acquire the license.

The remarkable communication system for emergency cases:

So now that I've given you a few alternatives that you can pick, here I am going to tell you about various other alternatives as well.

Ham transistor is the go-to correspondence framework to be used for basically every emergency system and it is the thing that MARS and ARES both use.

One of the pleasant effects is that a considerable measure of ham transistors can achieve the frequencies of national climate framework. That implies that in case you possess a radio, you can discover what's happening in the range.

Here is an underprivileged of alternative transistor frequencies which you ought to remember when both searching for radios and thinking of your emergency correspondences systems. Just to mollify all the know-it-alls who continue letting you know this rundown is really effective in light of the fact that you can't transmit on them. You should remember that they're valuable to screen in crises regardless of the fact that you can't send anything out, and I needed to make as complete a list as I can make for everybody.

FRS walkie-talkies

FRS radios or family radio service is an intense however short-extended service that you can use to speak with your family within your home or campground. This is a decent choice to add on your emergency survival pack since it is cheap and simple to make use of which implies that, everybody in your group or family can make use of it. FRS radios can likewise speak with GMRS that is General versatile radio service, as they share a few frequencies.

However, FRS two-way radios have their constraints to within its reach extraordinarily. Despite the fact that tests demonstrated that FRS radios can achieve a score of 22 to 36 miles, this is just feasible during ideal conditions which are extremely troublesome during calamities and emergency situation. So FRS radios are best to make use of the place inside your camp, it is still best to make use of all the more effective radios like HAM to get more range and a higher shot of external communication.

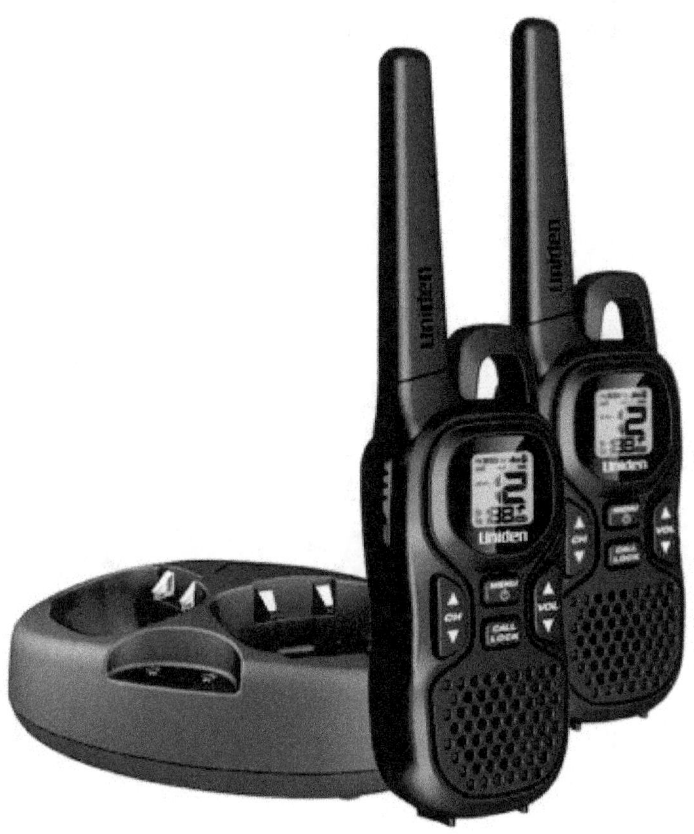

Scanner Radios

A scanner radio is one of the must have radios in your emergency survival kit as it gives you the capacity to listen to other radio transmissions in your general vicinity from various companies like fire divisions, police, emergency vehicle services, government offices, and air. Having a scanner radio during a trip is one of the ideal approaches to reach the world so you may know how to suitably react to the circumstance and for communicating with your family.

Chapter 3 – Survival communication tips

It is true without any doubt that the survival kit will work as the main thing which will make you survived from any of the problems which come to you. The need of survival kits for any family is different as all the families are having different sets of needs which are associated with them. If you want to get ready for any type of emergency situation then this survival kit will also help you in all situation.

Also, when you opt for having survival kits for any of the emergency circumstances which you face, you will also get the option of storing water and its purification tool. It may sometimes happen that you may need some kit which can be personalized by you. So, you can also customize the kit as per you desire without facing any kind of problem.

A proper plan of action along with your customized or even the essential survival kit will help you a lot in surviving from the tough situations along with the assistance to have an adequate supply of water with you as well, as water is a necessary and basic need for keep moving the vehicle of your life.

So many people are of the view that they will not face anything bad so there is no need of having any survival kit with them. But I must tell you here, that this thing is worst to be taken in mind owing to the fact that when it comes to survival, no one knees whenever you will get to need it at any time. It is also a matter of fact that no one can ever be able to get himself prepared for some kind of emergency situation but it is really better to think about to be safe before facing any kind of problem.

The contents which are going to be included in any of the survival kits vary from one place to another. Also, the purpose and location where the survival kit is going to be used will also determine what will be those contents, which are going to be included in that kit.

But, as far as the universality of the survival communication toolkit is concerned, there are some of the contents which are common to all the kits and which are necessary for survival in any kind of situation no matter how severe the situation are. So, you should be very careful about all the things which are common and also, do not forget to keep in mind the extent to which the survival kits may vary from one place to another.

So, just before making your own survival kit, you must be having in your mind about the tools which should be there in order to make your kit completed. You are required to take the proper communication tools with you along with other things which are required. If you are on an outside trip at some place which is at a forest or any mountains, your survival kit must be having some tools, which will help you to stay safe and secure when you are on your journey. You must be having a knife and an ax with you so that you can cut the branches of trees or anything which you require. This will help you in building your shed or any shelter so that you may become able to be secure and safe even if the weather conditions are not so good.

Now, it is not necessary that you should have the knife which is being made by the traditional ways. Anything which can be used as a sharpening tool can be taken as something which resembles knife and which will help you in cutting anything you want. For example, if you are having something to be called as canned food in your survival kit, but you must require having some sharp thing which can be used to cut the can. So, a knife or some sharp thing is a must thing which you require. Along with the cans of tin, the glass and some other things of the same hard material also require having something like a knife to be cut down.

Some more survival communication tips

Repeaters

There are a ton of repeaters in the world that can help you transmit long separations with only a radio. Essentially, a repeater will listen to the small radios in its quick surroundings and afterward impact the sign out for hundreds, or thousands, of miles. Clearly the repeaters should have got the capacity to do this, however, individuals who have repeaters are for the most part upon emergency communication and will have systems for reinforcement power as well.

There are even repeaters that make use of the internet. So in case, you take advantage of a repeater and have been struck in another location, then what you say on your minimal radio will impact out to that point on the opposite side of the world.

Utilizing stealth to work with a novice radio

Since ham radio individuals are cunning parcel and some spots don't permit the use of reception tools, there is an entire sub-sort of approaches to make the receiving wires so they can't be identified. Receiving wires can be made out of flagpoles, stepping stools, wall, railings, and a considerable measure of different things on display. They can likewise be covered up with some other internal things or covers.

The Ham radio group

As I've said, novice radio services are not just innovative and clever, they're extremely tuned in to taking care of the emergency situation. There are a few groups that make use of a ham radio for managing trips or for inquiry and salvage. The greater of the two are Radio Amateur Civil Emergency Service (RACES) and Amateur Radio Emergency Service (ARES).

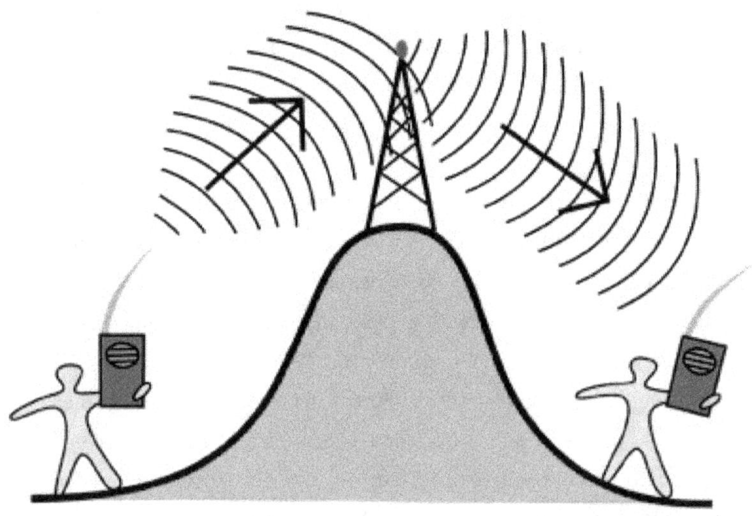

In case you need to start finding out about ham radio as a viable emergency communications framework for you or your family, look at the Prepared Ham Forum. Heaps of accommodating individuals will also be there to assist you in any kind of emergency situation.

Inventive approaches to speak with ham frequencies

With the right gear and some practice, you can undoubtedly get far and wide. What's more, you don't need to really purchase a radio to do it. That is the biggest aspect regarding learning and utilizing ham radio. You can actually make a working radio out of scrap. There will dependably be a scrap. You will dependably have the capacity to make a radio.

Notwithstanding the plenty of ham radio hardware and data accessible, a great premise of the hypothesis can make them converse with individuals regardless of the possibility that all power and gadgets are taken out. Here are a few case of what you can do with a small information.

In the case of a helicopter protection, most pilots will attempt to have land as a first choice. If a sufficiently extensive clearing is accessible than adequate size will rely on the ground, height, wind conditions, and ability of the pilot, a clearing of no less than 80 feet is the thing that generally require. Attempt and position yourself with your back to the wind-confronting the clearing so you're at the 12 to 3 clock position. After it lands, sit tight for salvage workforce to come to you, don't head out to the helicopter, when force is diminished, the rotors can wind up brought down to a point where they can execute a normal tallness individual particularly in case you are up at the slope of the helicopter.

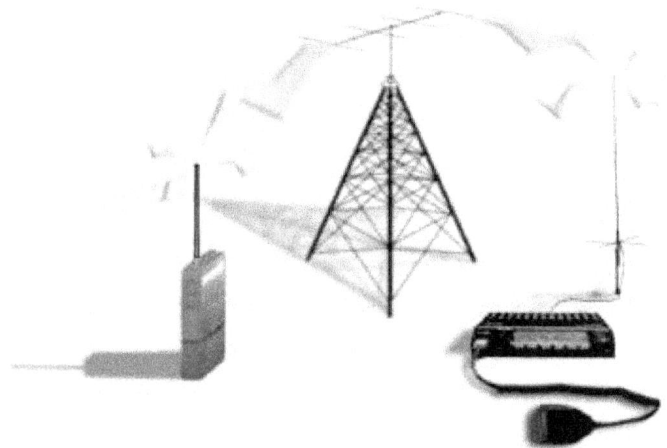

Since weight influences fuel limit which thus influences range and time of flight, don't hope to take your pack or tool with you. In the occasion, the group chooses to bring down a crane or bushel, by and large, a rescuer will ride it down. Try not to attempt and help, particularly abstain from attempting to get the crate or link before it has an opportunity to touch the ground at any rate. The rotors can get the electricity produced via friction over long separations and touching a link or wicker bin before it grounds can give you a stun.

Chapter 4 – How to get rescued by survival communication?

Calling for help or getting protected in an emergency situation is not something the vast majority of us need to do. But rather by investing enough energy outside will give you chances that are you'll encounter some sort of emergency. With regards to making use of your mobile phone and getting safeguarded, here are the tips you can take after, that will help rescuers discover you rapidly, help them, and get you out securely. A snappy salvage expands the chances of survival and can lessen the introduction to safeguarding the parties. Communication and flagging assume an essential part in proficient wild protects. Here are a few things to be considered.

Telling somebody about your plan is imperative. Before you leave for your trip, let somebody know your normal return time, trail or course, destination, auto type and plate number, fundamental tools you'll have, your mobile phone number and bearer, and different names and data related to you. At times, you can likewise portray the color of your tent and coat, and rundown supplies.

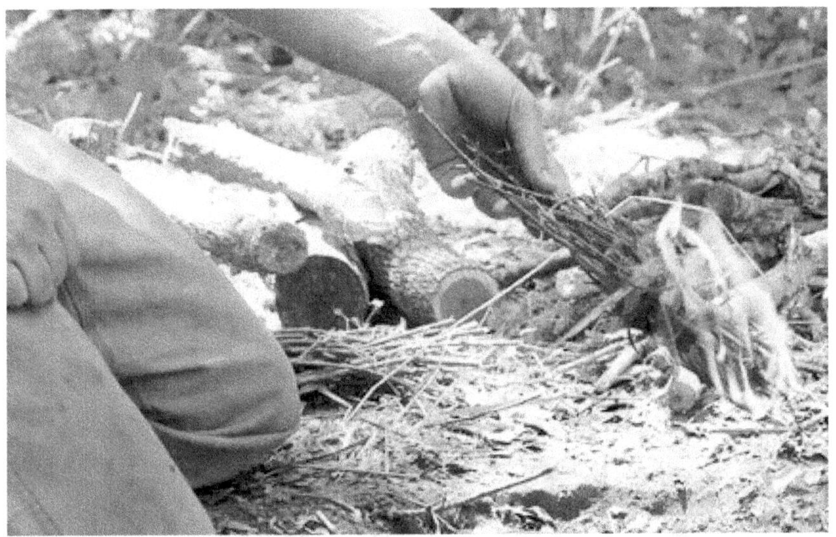

Although, some spots won't have a mobile network accessible in the far off places, the scope is expanding and in so many situations of crises, mobile phones are the most widely recognized method for starting salvage for climbers and explorers. You ought to switch off your phone or radio in case you have one to monitor batteries till you are prepared to make use of it. In cool situations attempt and keep your communication tool near your body to keep it warm and also to preserve the battery life between layers of clothing items. Most new phones consequently settle your area when you make an emergency call, this isn't generally ensured and you can find a way to offer assistance.

A. Prior to your excursion initiate your phones programmed area setting which empowers E911 to ascertain your position.

B. Turn on your phone once per day before an emergency for around 5 minutes, when fueled up phones check in with the closest tower. This should be done regardless of the fact that there is an insufficient sign to make a call, it can be sufficient to leave an electronic trail.

C. Radios and most mobile phones work disconnected from the net of site significance, for example, slopes, mountains, or overwhelming tree spread can obstruct the signals. Satellite phones require an unhindered perspective of the sky. To make an emergency call, higher open areas will give the best flag. So you are required to hold your phone at a manageable distance and pivot around to locate the best group. When you locate the best spot, come back to that spot for future calls.

- Consider what data you'll have to pass on to the emergency service provider. Dial the number of the emergency individual before your emergency contact. Stay quiet, at the request, express your name, your area with however many subtle elements as can be allowed.

- In case, you don't have the foggiest idea about your area depicting encompassing area elements then last known unmistakable focus on the area will likewise offer assistance. Let them know your emergency and individuals included, type of hardware, the amount of food items and fuel you have and the color of the tent, rucksack, garments, and so on, including your emergency contacts data.

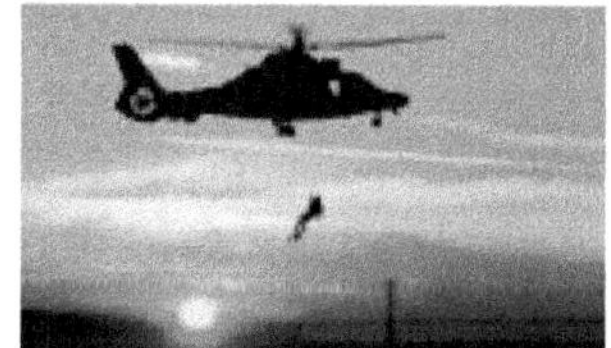

Notice your plan of activity stay put, attempt and exit, set up portable shelter, and assemble a fire, and so on. Before hanging up, let them know you'll turn off your phone and play Judas five minutes before, then look for the highest point of consistently or two, unless told generally by the 911 administrator. Take after some other directions that have been given.

- In case you don't have enough groups to support but a spotty sign, it's conceivable to get an instant message out regardless of the possibility that you can't get a call through. Most emergency services aren't set up to get instant messages so make use of your emergency contact. In case you benefited an occupation of pre-outing communication you'll have the capacity to keep your content short, they'll know who it's originating from and right now have fundamental data.

To flag others material can be regular and you can make use of sticks, rocks, soil, shadows, manmade garments, packs, tents, space covers or both. The vital thing to recall is to take after the class standard for ground to Air signals. "C" remains for Contrast, you perform this with shading that differences the environment. This can be a dark shadow against white snow which can be done by borrowing a trench or Orange tent over green vegetation. The "L" remains for the area, you need an open range that can be seen from various bearings and is near to your own zone.

"A" stands for Angularity, the straighter your lines and more honed your corners are, the better it is. There are not many common 90 degree corners in nature so having them in a sign will get a rescuers attention. "S" remains for Size, the greater your sign the better. S remains for shape, there aren't an excessive number of straight corners or 90-degree twists in nature so having a sign with straight lines and sharp corners will emerge more. The state of your sign can likewise convey data to an air group. A huge implies that you require help. The later X tells the team that you have been harmed, and then you can make use of vast bolts to impart the bearing of travel in case you're leaving a signed zone.

- Development additionally gets the attention, you can perform this with lively arm waves or a shirt toward the end of a shaft. The shirt will likewise have the advantage of informing the helicopter group of the heading of the wind as they have to confront into the wind to make a lift for landing and taking off. A legitimate work makes use of sign mirror that will be spotted to about 100 miles.

- Space covers, aluminum foil, watches, and anything which sparkles can likewise be made out of it. During the evening flares, headlamp (light), and chemical sticks work best. Three sign are light and simple to pack are a sign mirror, shriek, and compound stick. Different things can likewise work assign materials.

Fire signs are one of the best strategies for flagging salvage. The two fundamental issues are bringing on woods fires and the time window between getting the fire to deliver enough smoke to be seen and airship passing. Care must be taken to clear the encompassing vegetation and set up the ground for a fire. Another issue can be the individuals who do not distinguish the fire as a sign.

To fabricate a sign fire, you should first set up the site. Locate an open area near your camp or where you'll invest the majority of your energy. Clear the fire zone, scratching the ground to exposed earth, and broaden it out no less than 15 feet. Prep the kindling with every phase of wood put in a log lodge design with small pieces at the base and bigger wood toward the top.

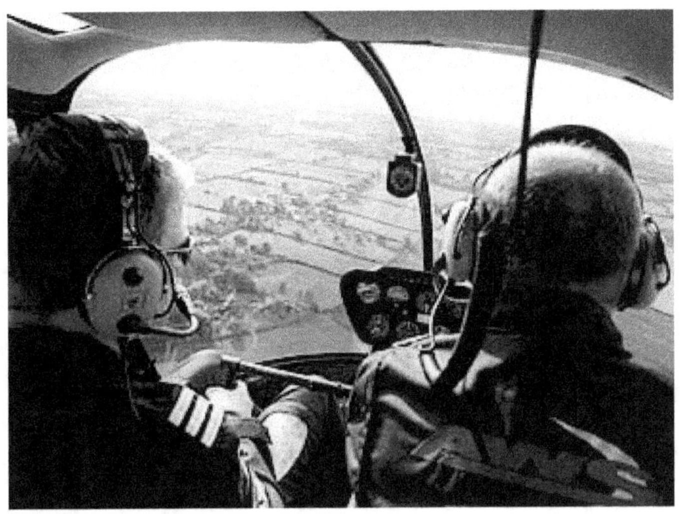

Close to the top you ought to have one to three feet of fuel, and green material including pine limbs, branches, grass, leaves. It creates more smoke than dead dry material. The fire burning material and fuel ought to be dry and dead. Having the green stuff on top will keep the kindling dry at the base. Have a tender close-by and keep dry. When you first hear an airplane or realize that safeguard is in the general zone or fast approaching begin the fire. Once you have waist high flares add green material as expected to keep delivering the smoke.

Conclusion

It is really a matter of fact that everyone feels contented and secure in one's own house. No one is willing to leave one's home or no one will want to have a home which is not protected by the security locks and other things like this. No one will really want to have his/her family in an unprotected environment where there are no locks on the door. It is just like as if you are not having the survival kit with you when you need it the most no matter wherever you are. God forbade, if any of the natural tragedy comes, then your essential survival kit will definitely help you in surviving even in a bad situation. Survival communication comes out to be necessary when you are at trip or may be when you are facing a critical situation.

Survival Cookbook

Introduction

Are you preparing yourself for the most unfavorable circumstances? What would happen if a natural disaster strikes down and you're left alone with very little to carry on? For this very reason, you have to be prepared. If you are a professional prepper, this book is just right for you. Just add this book to your prepping stuff and you'd be able to survive all the tough conditions.

The recipes given in this book are simple and really easy to understand. In times where you have to survive and fight a battle against catastrophes, this book would help you feel like home. These recipes are not only easy and just what a prepper needs, they are really delicious too. You'd not feel you have a survival problem.

In this book, I am sharing 20 recipes that are tasty and what is the best thing about these recipes is that they can be kept in a mason jar for longer periods of time. For, who knows how long you will have to survive and how long would it take someone to come at your rescue. The food that you'd make using these recipes could be preserved and kept for times you have nothing to eat to keep your life going.

Doing the Stuff of confidence requires significant investment, assets, tools, and other things as well. More critical than any of these is the action you take. With just twenty four hours in a day, you can't generally trek to your own space in the forested areas to practice wild basic instincts. Tumultuous calendars and time requirements consume your accessibility. There is no better approach to hang out with your friends and family than to acquaint them with outside independence abilities in a controlled setting.

I have chosen these recipes that are to be made in mason jars because in times where you're alone and you need to survive, you should be able to preserve food for long. Because you are not sure when help would come and it might even take a long period of time before you are rescued so you have to be sure you have preserved enough food for a long period of time.

The capacity to make fire under any condition is basic thing to be done during survival. With How to Build a prepping there are numerous systems to assemble a fire; a fire drill, seething plants and trees, daylight, striking shake that contains iron, for example, rock, and obviously matches and lighters. Fire craft is the capacity to make, control, and utilize fire to help in one's survival. Another basic aptitude in Prepping is the capacity to transfer fire, normally via burning or heating coal in some type of dry sage grass to keep it seething.

There are a total of 20 recipes that you'd learn to make which can be preserved and kept for future use. For when you have to survive, it is not just the present you should be worried about, the future should be taken care of too.

Chapter 1 – Survival Food Storage

If you are a want to-be survivor or a prepper and you have no idea where to start, I'll guide you through that in this chapter. Before anything, the first thing you should do is to store food. Because to make use of the 20 recipes that I've shared in this book, you have to be sure you have almost everything that you need with you and the amount of all that should also be enough to keep you going for a long time. Getting better prepped for unfavorable circumstances doesn't mean you're a pessimist. It means that you're wise and you are thinking about your family and your survival in adverse conditions for who knows when could that happen? So, where to start with storing enough food to help you survive for a long while.

Survival tips envelop a few primitive aptitudes to shape your general surroundings and meet your survival needs. Recall, prepping shows you how to do every one of different things with only a basic tool and the learning in your mind. Each of these prepping aptitudes have numerous littler subsets of undertakings and capacities that make them up.

As should be obvious there is a long way to go. While turning into a prepping expert can take quite a while and without any doubt, there are so many little abilities that can be immediately figured out how to kick you off. Moreover, a part of the more basic abilities like making cordage and branches have numerous uses and can be connected to more than one control. At it is the most basic level of prepping, here is the specialty of going out into the forested areas and getting by just with the clothes on your back and an edged tool. About each ability and most prepping activities utilize a prepping device to make your work simpler.

Steps involved in storing survival food

Let's have a look at how you can store enough amount of food to help you survive before the circumstances come back to normal,

1.   Planning:

First thing to do anything is to plan. You cannot just go on and start doing something. You have to make a plan first. This is not the easiest of all the steps. Going to the market and buying stuff is easier but what to buy and in what quantity and from where etc. these require certain decisions to be made. This step is mostly ignore but trust me, you want to do this. So planning is the first and the most critical step involved in storing food.

2.   Buying:

So after you've made a plan, go out there and start buying. This should be simple. Get a list of food items to buy, grab your wallet and drive to the market and buy all the stuff.

3.   Preserving:

The third step is to preserve food. This step is really important. Now you have to make sure that you preserve the food long enough so that it can be eaten when you want to eat it. Try to get things that can be preserved for at least three years.

4.   Organizing:

This is really important that you keep all the food in an organized way. Keep everything separate and in an orderly manner in the storage room.

5. Eating:

This is the best part, of course. For this I've 20 really good recipes for you in the upcoming chapters of this book. You would love each and every recipe.

Now that you have known what are the steps you need to take to store food for prepping. Now let's take a look at how you can store different food items.

6. Canning:

This is a traditional method to preserve food for long periods of times. This involves partially cooking the food to kill any germs or bacteria, adding additives like sugar syrup etc. cleaning the cans or glass jars, drying them and filling them with the food items and then sealing them to store for a long period of time.

7. Drying:

This is probably the easiest way of preserving food. This requires no real efforts. It is known that bacteria and mold grow in moisture. So rest assured, you could keep the food you dry for long span of time and without fearing that it will rot or catch bacteria.

8. *Salt curing:*

This is an old method which was used to preserve meat for long time. Salt helps keep the meat safe from bacteria because bacteria cannot survive more than 10% of concentration of salt in something. You can rub a mixture of sugar and salt on meat and keep it tightly shut in a pot or jar and keeping it somewhere the temperature is cool.

9. *Refrigeration:*

This the very famous and very common way of preserving food. Keeping beef, mutton, poultry, cooked food and other items in a refrigerator keeps them safe for a long period of time by keeping the food frozen or cold.

Chapter 2 – 10 Delicious Prepping Recipes for All Seasons in Mason Jars

You have everything kept in your storage to help you survive during circumstances that are adverse. Now you'd need some recipes that would make you feel normal and happy even in times of distress. Let's have a look at some of these recipes,

1) ALMOND MILK & HONEY PORRIDGE:

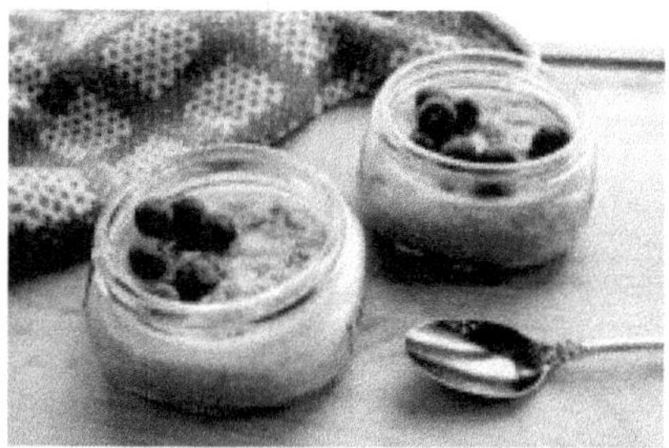

http://photos2.demandstudios.com/DM-Resize/www.livestrong.com/ls_images/recipes/00000/45/77/0/almond-milk-honey-porridge-17754.jpg?w=280&h=280&keep_ratio=1

This is a very simple but nutritious and satisfying recipe that you would be able to make in just 15 minutes. This recipe would serve 3 persons. You would need the following ingredients,

- Cooked Quinoa (2 cups)

- Ground Nutmeg (2 pinches)

- Unsweetened almond milk (1 and a half cup)

- Natural Almond Butter (1 and half tbsp.)

- Vanilla extract (1 and half tbsp.)

- Sea Salt (1 pinch)

What to do?

1. Blend quinoa and one cup almond milk in a blender until mixed well. Pour this mixture in a pot and cook over medium heat. Take the remaining half cup of almond milk and mix it in the mixture using a stirrer. Add vanilla essence, nutmeg and sea salt into the mixture and cook until bubbles start appearing. Add almond butter and stir.

2. Take mason jars and pour the mixture into them and garnish them with fresh berries if you like.

2) CHICKEN CURRY SALAD WITH GREENS:

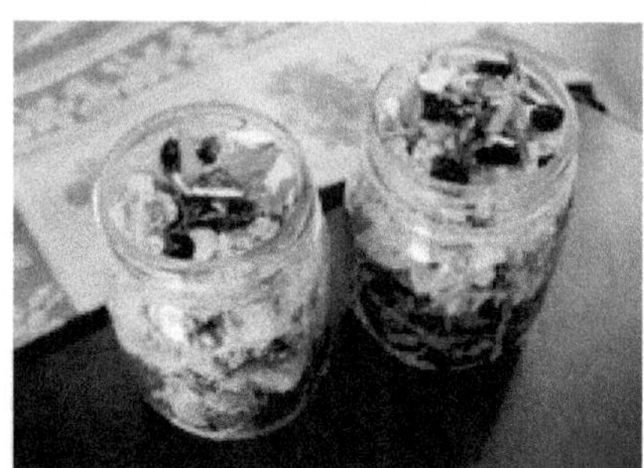

http://photos2.demandstudios.com/DM-Resize/www.livestrong.com/ls_images/recipes/00000/55/77/0/chicken-curry-salad-greens-17755.jpg?w=280&h=280&keep_ratio=1

This is a creamy chicken salad that is a very good source of protein for your body. It would take almost an hour for you to complete this recipe. This recipe serves 7 people. The ingredients are,

- Skinless Chicken Breast (3 pieces)

- Mayonnaise (1/3 cup)

- Low-fat Greek yogurt (1/3 cup)

- Curry Powder (1 serving)

- Sea salt (half tsp)

- Ground Black Pepper (1 dash)

- 1 Grated carrot

- 1 chopped celery stalk

- Raisins (1/2 cup)

- Unsalted Dry Toasted Slivered Almonds (1/4 cup)

- Arugula (4 cups)

What to do?

- Preheat your oven at 375 degrees. Take a large baking tray and cover it with tinfoil. Bake the chicken in the over for almost 45 minutes. The chicken should be thoroughly cooked and light golden brown in color. Let it cool down for some time. Take the chicken and shred the meat.

- Whisk mayo, Greek yogurt, salt and pepper in a small bowl. Add 1 tbsp.. of curry powder to the mixture and mix it well. You can add more curry powder according to your taste.

- Take a bowl and put the shredded chicken, grated carrot and chopped celery in it. Pour the curry sauce that you've made into the bowl and mix everything gently. Put raisins and almonds in the mixture too. Take a mason jar and make a layer of arugula at the bottom and then pour the curry salad above it. Your recipe is ready!

3) FRUIT SOUP WITH TOASTED NUTS:

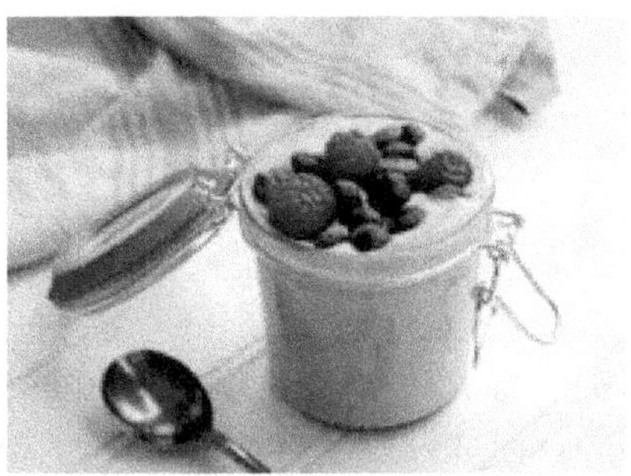

http://photos2.demandstudios.com/DM-Resize/www.livestrong.com/
ls_images/recipes/00000/16/77/0/fruit-soup-toasted-nuts-17761.jpg?
w=280&h=280&keep_ratio=1

This recipe is full of tasty Greek yogurt combined with fruit. This recipe is perfect for a strong protein breakfast. Takes just 15 minutes to make and serves 2 people. The ingredients include,

- Shelled Pistachios (2 tbsp.)

- low-fat Greek yogurt (1 and a half cup)

- Frozen Mixed Berries Frozen (1 cup)

- Vanilla extract (1 1/4 tsp)

- Agave nectar (2 tbsp.)

- Ground nutmeg (1 pinch)

- Unsweetened Almond Milk (1/2 cup)

- Raspberries (1/4 cup)

What to do?

If you want you can roast the nuts at 350 degrees for 5 minutes. Take Greek yogurt, berries, vanilla, and agave nectar, nutmeg and almond milk and blend them well in a blender. Make sure the result is creamy and smooth. Store in a Mason jar and put lots of fruit on top of it. Serve with a spoon when you want to eat.

4) CHICKEN APPLE AND CASHEW SALAD:

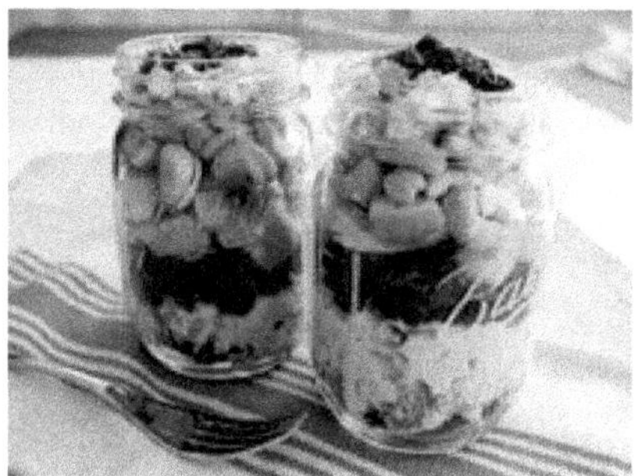

http://photos2.demandstudios.com/DM-Resize/www.livestrong.com/
ls_images/recipes/00000/85/77/0/chicken-apple-cashew-salad-17758.jpg?
w=280&h=280&keep_ratio=1

A perfect balanced lunch with carbohydrates, proteins and fat. This recipe would take an hour to make and will serve 8 people. Following are the ingredients,

- Skinless Chicken Breast (3 pieces)

- Mayonnaise (1/3 cup)

- Low-fat Greek yogurt (1/3 cup)

- A medium celery stalk

- Sea Salt (1/2 tsp)

- Ground Black Pepper

- Chopped fresh Thyme (1/2 tsp)

- Chopped Green Apple (3 serving)

- Dry Roasted Unsalted Cashews (1/4 cup)

- Dried Cranberries (1/3 cup)

What to do?

- Preheat your oven at 375 degrees. Take a large baking tray and cover it with tinfoil. Bake the chicken in the over for almost 45 minutes. The chicken should be thoroughly cooked and light golden brown in color. Let it cool down for some time. Take the chicken and shred the meat.

- Whisk mayo, Greek yogurt, salt and pepper in a small bowl. Put in celery, celery leaves and thyme and stir well.

- Take a mason jar and make a layer of arugula at the bottom and then pour the chicken salad above it. Put green apple, cashews and cranberries on top. Enjoy!

5) OVERNIGHT APPLE PIE PROTEIN OATS:

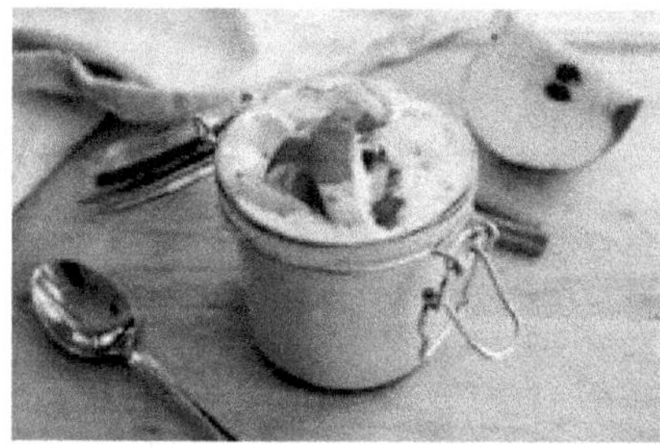

http://photos2.demandstudios.com/DM-Resize/www.livestrong.com/ls_images/recipes/00000/37/77/0/overnight-apple-pie-protein-oats-17773.jpg?w=280&h=280&keep_ratio=1

Another absolutely nutritious and yummy recipe. This recipe would take you 10 minutes to make. It serves 2 persons. You would need,

- 1 Second Cooking Spray

- Chopped apple (1 serving)

- Cinnamon (1 pinch)

- Proto Whey Vanilla (2 scoops)

- Low-fat Greek yogurt (2/3 cup)

- Vanilla extract (1 tsp)

- Ground Nutmeg (2 dash)

- Ground Allspice (2 dash)

- Sea Salt (1 pinch)

- Unsweetened Almond Milk (3/4 cup)

- Old Fashioned Oats (2/3 cup)

- Chia seeds (2 tbsp.)

What to do?

1. Take a small pan and spray it with cooking oil. Sauté apple until it's soft. Add cinnamon and set it aside.

2. Blend protein powder, Greek yogurt, and vanilla, nutmeg, and allspice, salt and almond milk in a blender until mixed well.

3. Mix the oats and chia seeds and stir them. Put them in mason jars.

4. Put sautéed apple on top of it. Stir it and keep it in the refrigerator overnight.

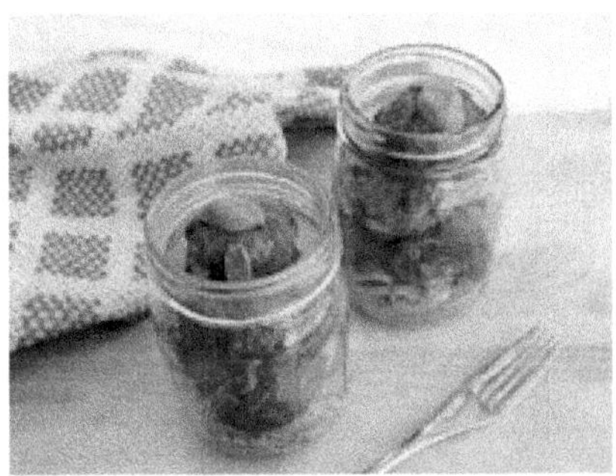

http://photos2.demandstudios.com/DM-Resize/www.livestrong.com/ls_images/recipes/00000/46/77/0/turkey-basil-meatballs-2-17764.jpg?w=280&h=280&keep_ratio=1

Meatballs are about fat and calories. A complete meal. This recipe would be complete in 50 minutes. Total servings: 6. let's check out the ingredients,

- 1 second Cooking Spray

- Grated onion (1/2)

- Minced garlic cloves (4)

- Fresh chopped Basil (1/4 cup)

- Beaten Egg (1)

- Worcestershire Sauce (1 tbsp.)

- All Natural Tomato Paste (2 tsp)

- Pecorino Grated Romano Cheese (4 tbsp.)

- Sea Salt (1/2 tsp)

- Pure Ground Black Pepper (1 serving)

- 92% lean Ground Turkey (20 oz)

- Gluten Free Bread Crumbs (1/3 cup)

- Organic Tomato Sauce (28 oz)

What to do?

1. Preheat your oven to 325 degrees. Take a large baking sheet and spray it with cooking spray.

2. Take a medium size bowl and whisk together onion, garlic, Worcestershire sauce, tomato paste, fresh basil, egg, cheese, salt and pepper until they are mixed well. Take the turkey and mix it with bread crumbs with your hands. Make sure you don't over-mix them. If the mixture is still wet, add some more bread crumbs.

3. Make 24 balls with your hands. Bake these balls for 20 minutes almost. Turn the balls halfway through the baking. Make sure you don't overcook the balls.

4. Meanwhile, make pasta according to the directions on the box.

5. Take a pot and heat the sauce in it over medium heat.

6. Make a layer of pasta in the Mason jar and put the meatballs and sauce above it. Garnish with basil.

7) UPSIDE DOWN CEREAL AND PROTEIN MILK:

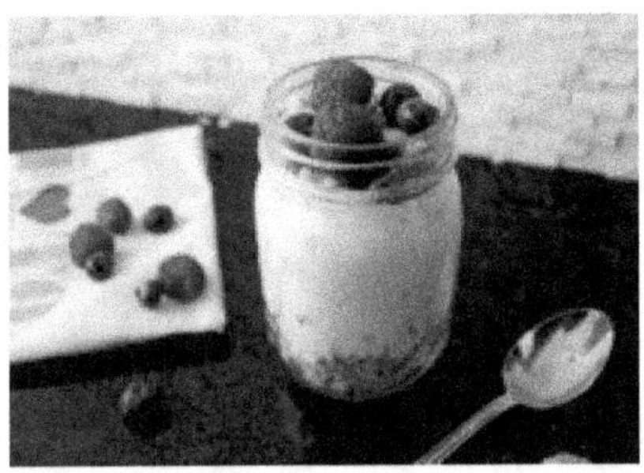

http://photos2.demandstudios.com/DM-Resize/www.livestrong.com/ ls_images/recipes/00000/26/77/0/upside-down-cereal-protein-milk-17762.jpg? w=280&h=280&keep_ratio=1

This recipe would help you boost up your metabolism. It would only take 5 minutes to be ready. Serves one person. The ingredients are,

- Gluten Free Sunrise Crunchy Vanilla (2/3 cup)

- Low-fat Greek yogurt (1 cup)

- Proto Whey, Vanilla Crème (1/2 scoops)

- Vanilla extract (1 tsp)

- Unsweetened Almond Milk (1/3 cup)

What to do?

1. Take a mason jar and pour cereal in it.

2. Blend Greek yogurt, protein powder, vanilla and almond milk in a blender until its smooth.

3. Before you serve it, pour protein milk on the cereal. Garnish it with fresh berries if you like.

8) BACON & EGGS IN A JAR:

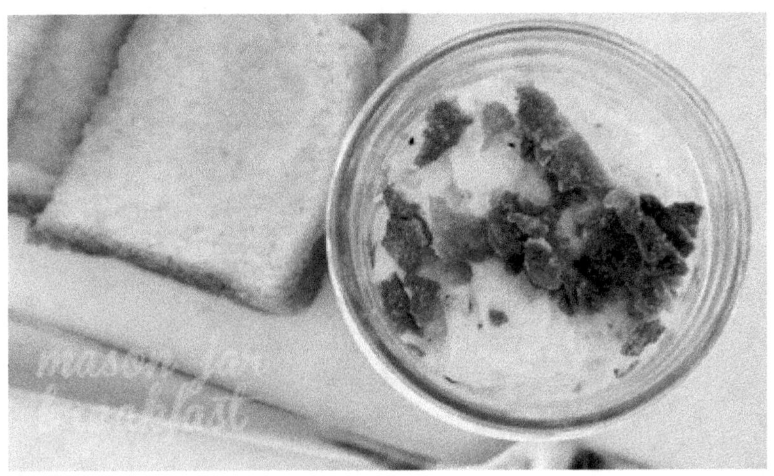

http://www.masonjarbreakfast.com/wp-content/uploads/2014/04/bacon-top.png

An instant recipe that would take only 5 minutes! The ingredients are,

- Bacon
- Eggs (2)
- Shredded Cheese
- Fresh Spinach
- Dash Salt & Pepper

What to do?

1. Take a bowl and mix eggs, spinach, salt & pepper and cheese together.

2. Take a mason jar and pour the mixture in it.

3. Cook the mixture in the microwave oven for 2 minutes at leasts.

4. Garnish with some additional cheese & bacon crumbles.

9) ACAI BANANA BERRY SMOOTHIE:

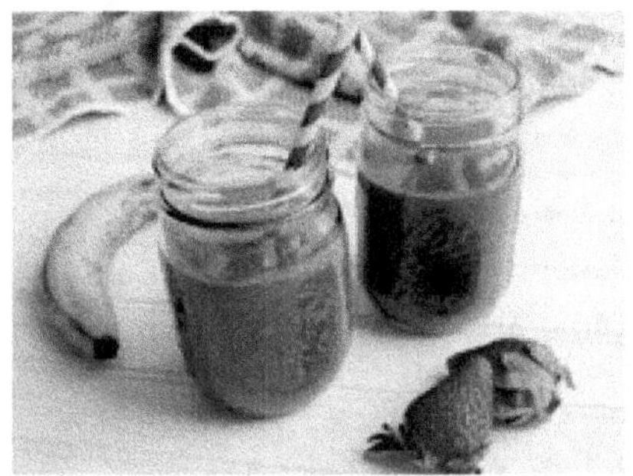

This smoothie is perfect for you when your blood sugar level drops. Takes 5 minutes to make, the ingredients include,

- Unsweetened almond milk (one and half cup)

- 1 Banana (medium)

- Chopped strawberries (1/2 cup)

- Acai powder (2 tbsp.)

- Proto Whey, Vanilla Cream (4 scoops)

What to do?

Take a blender and place almond milk, banana, strawberries, acai powder and Proto Whey Vanilla Cream in it until the mixture is blended completely. Add ice and blend until smooth and creamy.

10) SHRIMP AND VEGETABLE SALAD WITH COCONUT PEANUT SAUCE:

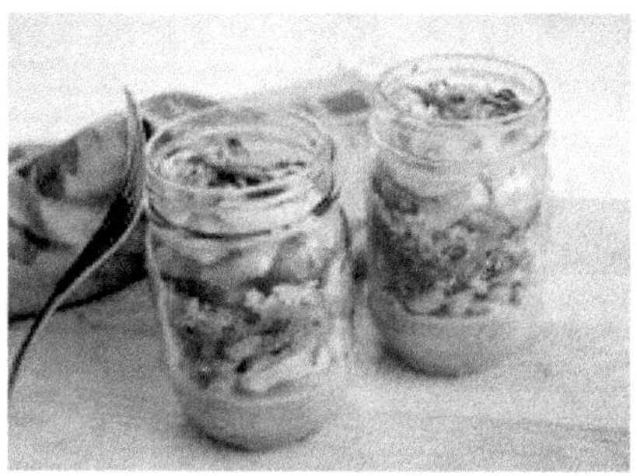

http://photos2.demandstudios.com/DM-Resize/www.livestrong.com/ls_images/recipes/00000/67/77/0/shrimp-vegetable-salad-coconut-peanut-sauce-17776.jpg?w=280&h=280&keep_ratio=1

This recipe would only take 25 minutes to make. Serves 4 people. The ingredients are,

- Light Coconut Milk Light (1/4 cup)

- All Natural Peanut Butter (1/4 cup)

- Low-sodium soy sauce (2 tbsp.)

- Agave nectar (1 tbsp.)

- Sriracha sauce (2 tsp)

- Minced garlic cloves (2)

- Raw Lime Juice (1 tbsp.)

- Cooked Medium Shrimp (16 oz)

- Organic Edamame (1 cup)

- 1 chopped red bell pepper

- 1 chopped yellow bell pepper

- 1 grated carrot

- Cooked Brown Basmati Rice (1 cup)

- Fresh chopped cilantro (1/4 cup)

What to do?

1. Whisk together the first 7 ingredients. Taste it and if you like you can add more lime juice.

2. Take a mason jar and layer it with coconut peanut sauce. Add shrimps, edamame, peppers, cilantro, carrots and brown rice on top

3. Shake the Mason jar when you want to eat it.

Chapter 3 – 10 Delicious Recipes for Summer in Mason Jars

In this chapter, I have 10 very nice recipes that you could make and eat all summers. Let's start!!

1) BLUEBERRY PANCAKE IN A JAR:

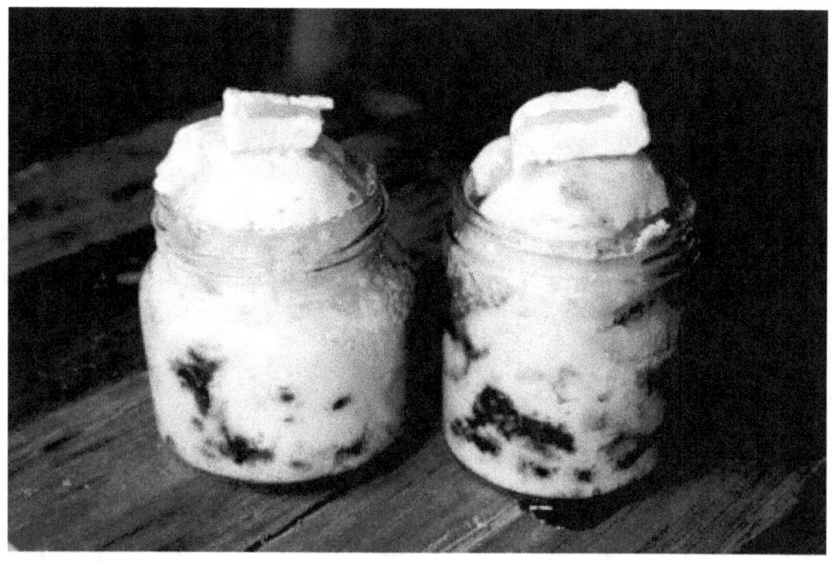

https://boyandtherabbit.files.wordpress.com/2012/07/blog-111.jpg?w=620

This is an incredible recipe for summers. You'll need the following ingredients,

- Flour (1 cup)

- Baking powder (1 tbsp.)

- Organic sugar (2 tbsp.)

- Melted vegan margarine (2 tbsp.)

- Nut milk (3/4 cup)

- Blueberries

What to do?

1. Take a small bowl and mix flour, baking powder and sugar in it. Add melted margarine and milk and stir.

2. Take mason jars and place blueberries at the bottom and fill the jars with the mixture. Pancake will rise after it's cooked. Microwave the jars for 1-1:30 minutes depending on the size of the jars. Let the jars cool. Then put margarine, blueberries and syrup on top. Enjoy!

2) STRAWBERRY & CHOCOLATE YOGURT PARFAIT:

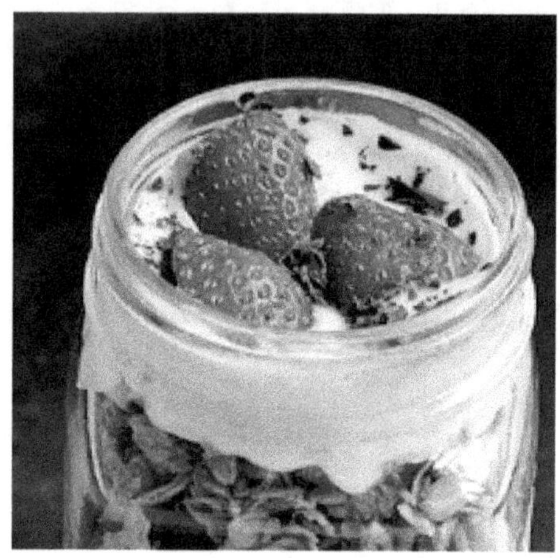

https://img.buzzfeed.com/buzzfeed-static/static/2014-07/7/18/enhanced/webdr10/grid-cell-32443-1404770627-20.jpg

- For this extremely delicious recipe, you'd need the following ingredients,

- Greek whole yogurt (1/2 - 3/4 cup)

- Granola (2/3 cup)

- 5-6 organic strawberries

- Organic chocolate bar (1-2 oz)

What to do?

1. Layer your parfait with 1/4 cup of yogurt.

2. Put 1/3 cup of granola on top.

3. Put pieces of chocolates and 2 strawberries sliced up on the top.

4. Repeat this procedure and put yogurt on top.

5. Garnish with strawberries and chocolate.

3) WHEAT BERRY APPLE SALAD:

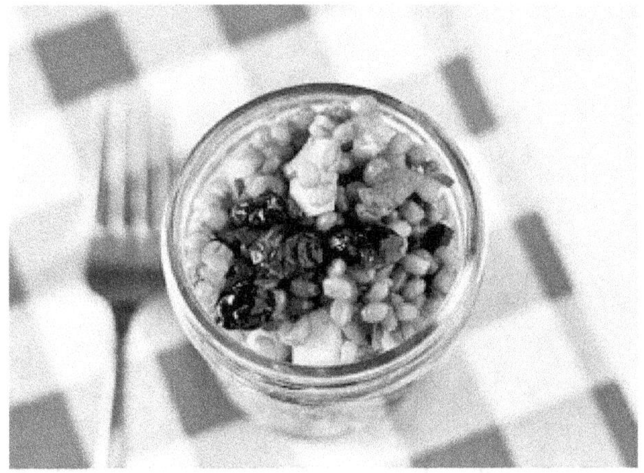

https://img.buzzfeed.com/buzzfeed-static/static/2014-07/7/18/enhanced/webdr06/grid-cell-20775-1404770869-29.jpg

Let's check out how you can make this yummy recipe,

- Wheat Berry Apple Salad

- Cooked wheat berries

- Chopped organic granny smith apple

- Dried cranberries

- Minced scallions or sweet onion

- Chopped Parsley

- Lemon juice

- Balsamic vinegar

- Olive oil

What to do?

Take all these ingredients and mix them in a bowl. Put the bowl aside. Take lemon juice, balsamic vinegar and olive oil in a bowl and whisk it until mixed completely. Mix these mixture with the salad.

4) SHRIMP FETA SALAD:

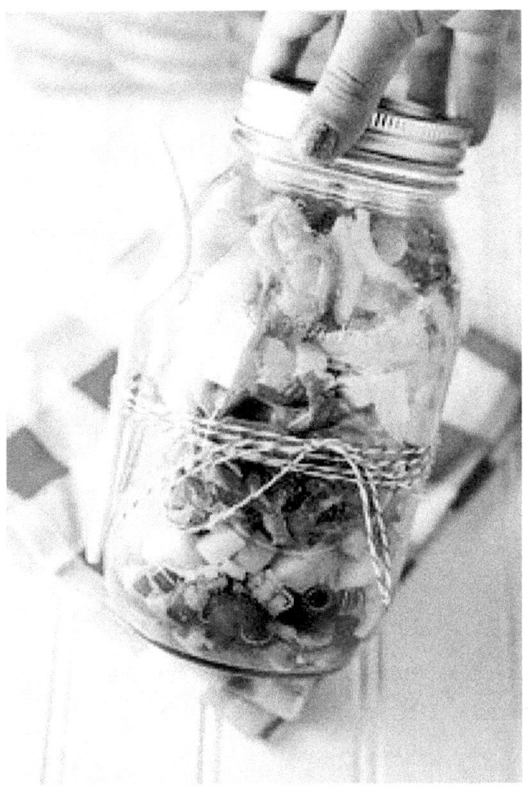

https://img.buzzfeed.com/buzzfeed-static/static/2014-07/7/18/enhanced/webdr06/grid-cell-25423-1404771284-7.jpg

This yummy summer salad would be a treat for you!

- Dressing of your liking

- Chopped avocado (2 tbsp.)

- 8 grape tomatoes

- Chopped red onion (1 tbsp.)

- Chopped cucumber (2 tbsp.)

- Romaine lettuce

- Baby spinach

- Chopped feta (2 tbsp.)

- 6-8 cooked shrimp

- 1 chopped boiled egg

- 2 slices of chopped cooked bacon

What to do?

Take a mason jar, make layers of all the above ingredients starting with the dressing of your own choice. Done!!

5) CAPRESE SALAD IN MASON JAR:

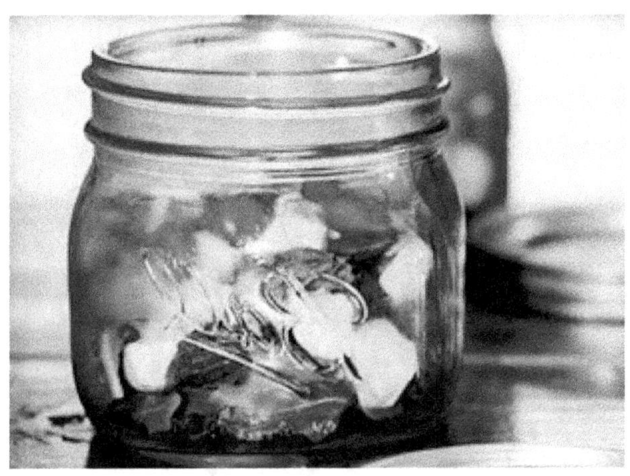

https://img.buzzfeed.com/buzzfeed-static/static/2014-07/7/18/enhanced/
webdr05/grid-cell-1507-1404771206-14.jpg

Ingredients for this recipe are,

- Arugula (2 cups)

- Green basil leaves only (1/2 cup)

- Purple basil leaves (1/2 cup)

- Cherry tomatoes (1/2 cup)

For the dressing:

- Olive oil (1/2 cup)

- Balsamic vinegar (1/2 tbsp.)

- Honey

- Maldon salt

- Black pepper (Cracked)

What to do?

1. Make layers of all the ingredients starting with arugula. Set the jars in the refrigerator to cool.

2. Whisk all the items for dressing.

3. Put the dressing on top of the salads.

4. Shake the jars before eating.

6) LEMON RASPBERRY MOUSSE PIE:

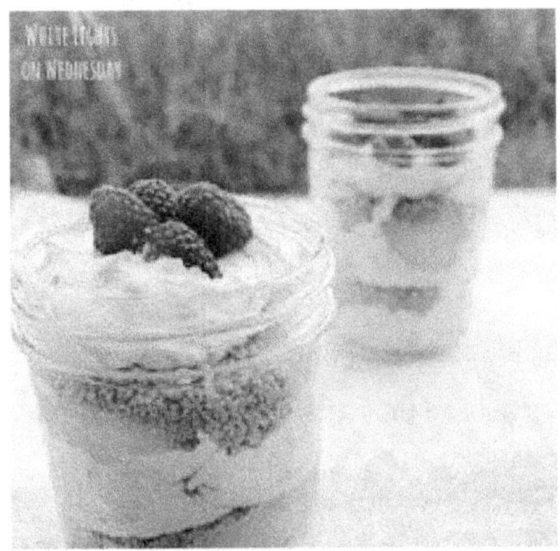

https://img.buzzfeed.com/buzzfeed-static/static/2014-07/7/19/enhanced/webdr06/grid-cell-396-1404774781-3.jpg

This is an excellent prepping recipe for summers. Let's take a look at the ingredients,

- Thawed Vanilla Cool Whip Topping, (1 tub)

- Lucky Leaf Red Raspberry Pie Filling (3/4 cup)

- Lucky Leaf Lemon Pie Filling (1/2 cup)

- Graham cracker crumbs (1 cup)

- Melted unsalted butter (2 tbsp.)

- Fresh raspberries (if you like)

What to do?

1. Take small bowl and mix Graham cracker crumbs and butter. Mix it really well.

2. Take a medium bowl, mix and fold thawed Cool Whip and red raspberry pie filling in it. Combine it well and then keep it a aside.

3. Take mason jars and put 2 tbsp. of graham cracker crumbs in the bottom. Put 1/2 cup raspberry mousse on it. Then top it with 2 tbsp. of lemon pie filling. Repeat all the steps.

4. Add raspberries on top.

7) ANTIPASTO SALAD IN A JAR:

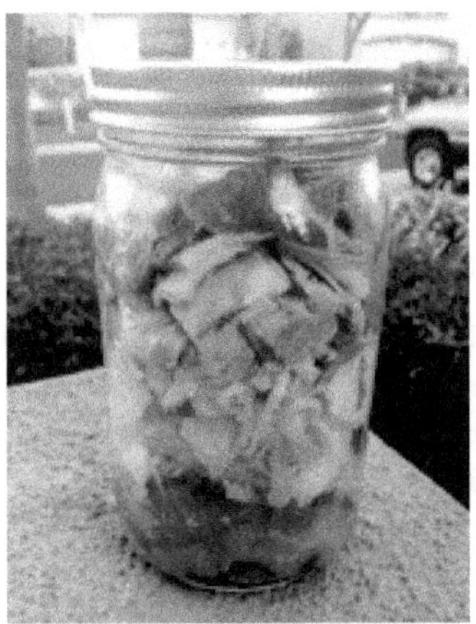

http://www.chaosandlove.com/wp-content/uploads/
2012/10/20121002-083712.jpg

This is a simple summer salad that is perfect for lunch. It's super fast. It would take only 20 minutes. Here are the ingredients,

- Salami, mortadella and capicola

- 1 head iceberg lettuce

- 4 Roma tomatoes

- Sliced pepperoncini (¼ cup)

- Sliced black olives (¼ cup)

- Olive oil (½ cup)

- Red wine vinegar (¼ cup)

- Salt and pepper

What to do?

1. Take a bowl and put oil, vinegar, salt and pepper in it and mix well.

2. Put tomatoes, pepperoncini and olives in it.

3. Take the meat and cut it in small pieces and put in the bowl with the mixture.

4. Fill the mason jars with this mixture.

5. Put lettuce on top.

6. Refrigerate the jars until you want to eat it.

8) STRAWBERRY AND GOAT CHEESE MASON JAR SALAD:

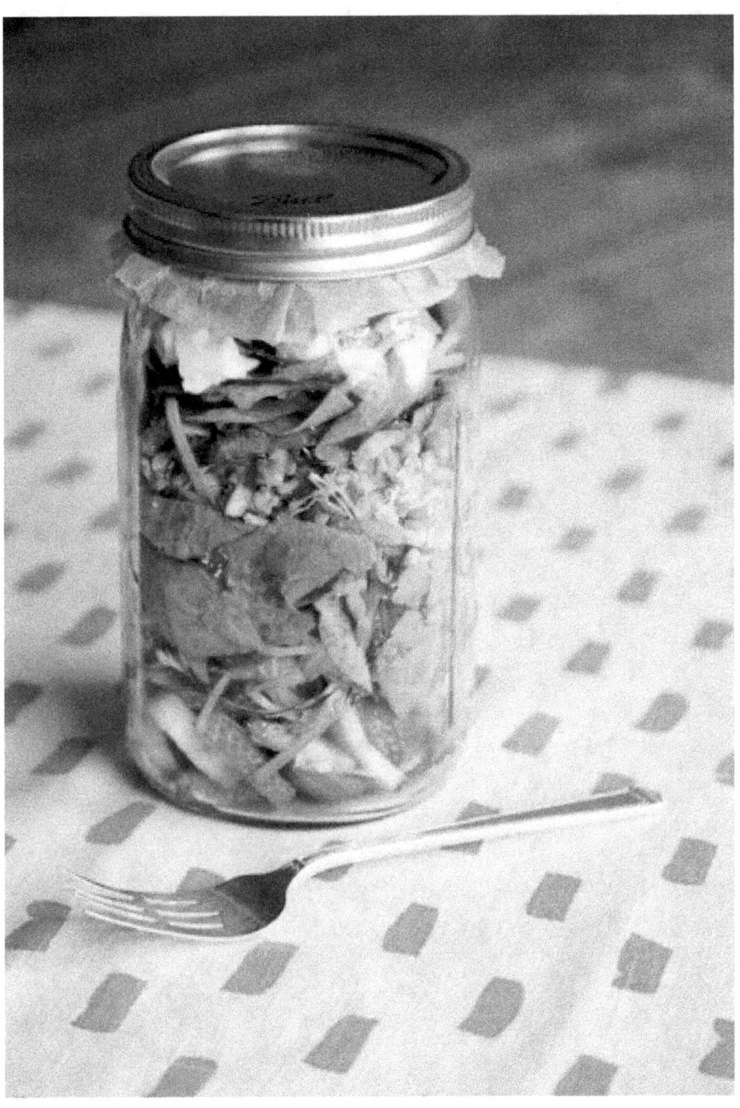

This recipe is really simple and really very yummy. This salad includes the following ingredients,

- Sliced strawberries (2/3 cup)

- Spinach leaves (3 cups)

- Chopped walnuts (3 cups)

- Crumbled goat cheese (1.5 ounces)

- Balsamic vinaigrette or blueberry vinaigrette (2-3 tbsp.)

What to do?

1. Take a mason jar and put strawberries in the bottom. Next put salad dressing. Spinach comes next and then walnuts. Add the remaining spinach and put goat cheese on the top.

2. Put the vinaigrette and then seal the jar. Refrigerate the salad.

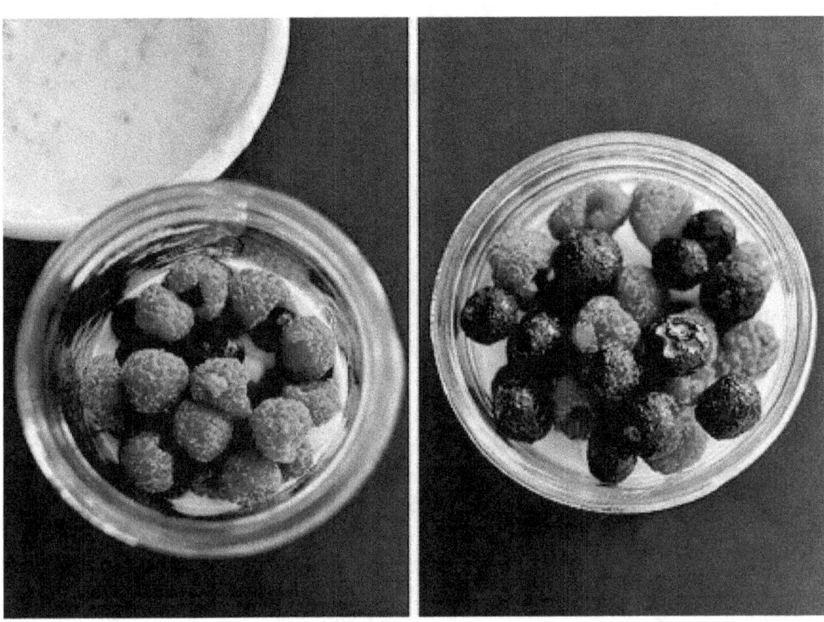

http://iowagirleats.com/2013/01/15/make-ahead-fruit-yogurt-breakfast-parfaits/makeaheadfruitandyogurtbreakfastparfaits_11_mini/

This is the perfect prepping recipe to cheer you up. Let's take a look at the ingredients,

- Uncooked certified gluten-free old fashioned oats (1/3 cup)

- Greek yogurt (6oz)

- Chia seeds (1 tsp)

- Milk (almond, cow, soy, etc.) (1 tbsp.)

- Frozen mixed fruit and berries (1 cup)

What to do?

1. Take a bowl and mix yogurt, oats, chia seeds, and milk in it.

2. Put a layer in Mason jar.

3. Add fruits and berries. Pour the remaining yogurt on top.

4. Garnish with berries.

5. Refrigerate until you're ready to eat.

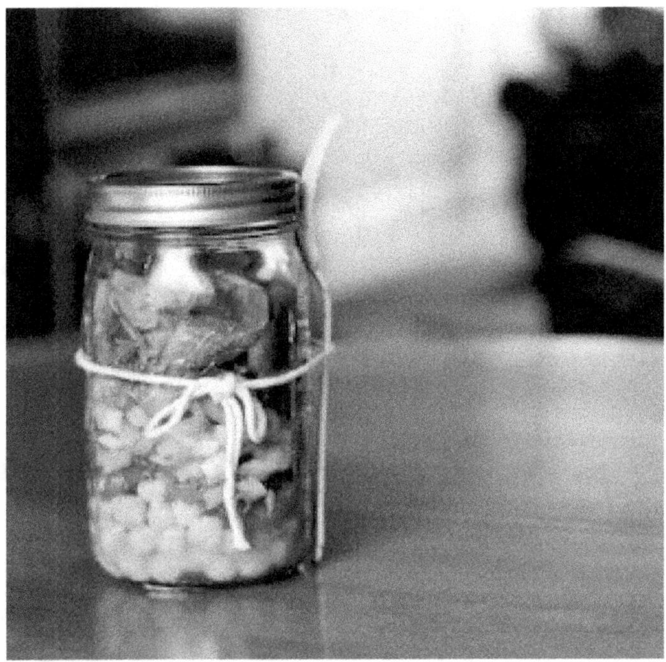

https://d3rgj9au57pk8c.cloudfront.net/uploaded/attachments/10803.jpg?v=befba6

This is another really simple salad that you can make in no time. A delight for you in summers. The items you need are,

- 2 tbsp. easy lemon vinaigrette (see below)

- Chickpeas (1 cup)

- sun-dried or oven roasted tomatoes (1/2 cup)

- Chopped Spring onion (1/4 cup)

- Chopped red onion (1/4 cup)

- Chopped olives (1/2 cup)

- Chopped piquillo peppers (1/4 cup)

- Fresh spinach (1/2 cup)

What to do?

Mix all the ingredients in a mason jar and refrigerate it until you're ready to eat.

Chapter 4 – What Food You Should Take During Prepping?

In this chapter, I would tell you what food you should keep and store during prepping. You don't want to miss anything that could be very healthy for you when you need it during unfavorable circumstances.

What food items should you store for prepping?

Now this is a hard decision because there are just so many things that you would to store. So make it easy for you, I'll ask you to store everything that you can. Not easy? It is if you have a list of everything you should store to help you survive when the circumstances take a very bad turn and you have to fight a surviving battle. Let's have a look at the list of everything that you should store for prepping,

Distilled water

Water is the most important thing that you'd need to survive in unfavorable conditions. You won't be able to make it for more than 3 days without water. So let's keep water on the top of the list of everything that you need to store. Make sure you've store plenty of water that is clean and pure.

Dehydrated powdered milk

Make sure you've bought enough powdered milk to keep in your storage.

Frozen dried eggs and powdered eggs

Buy frozen dried eggs and powdered eggs to keep in your storage. These eggs are 100% pure with no preservatives. Eggs usually last longer and don't need refrigeration.

Hard Cheese

To keep the cheese from rotting and catching bacteria, keep it stored in wax cases. This would keep the cheese from catching moisture too.

Protein bars and drinks

High in protein, protein bars and drinks are a must for your storage for they are a source of instant protein to your body.

Canned meat (Poultry, beef, mutton & seafood)

Meat is very important for human body. 90% of the sustenance required to survive is provided by meat. So make sure you save a lot of meat.

Coffee & tea

When you have to survive, it's essential that you stay alert. And for this you have to stock a lot of coffee and tea.

Essential cooking oils

To cook food, you'd need a lot oil. Make sure you stock a lot of oils in your storage. Stock olive oil, coconut oil, ghee, butter, lard and other essential oils.

Whole wheat flour

Stock a lot of wheat flour in your storage. A lot. Because you'll be needing wheat flour in a lot of your dishes.

1. Cereals, rice, corn etc.

2. Cornmeal, oats and oatmeal

3. Bread, crackers, pastas etc.

4. Jams and Jellies

5. Nuts, raisins, seeds etc.

6. Iodized salt

7. Sugar

8. Herbs and spices

9. Canned fruits and vegetables

10. Honey

11. Different sauces, vinegar

Make sure you get everything in enough quantities to keep in your storage room for prepping. If you feel like adding some other things that you want in this list, go on and do that.

Conclusion

One thing that is to be kept in mind when you prep is that you should not solely focus on food. Make sure you have other things with you too. You should have different medications, first-aid kits, enough amount of water to drink and to use for other purposes. Make sure you have everything you could need when the times are tough and adverse.

The recipes given in this book look fancy and flashy but they are really simple and really useful. You would not feel the severity of the circumstances if you are able to master some of these prepping recipes. You don't want to be thinking about how adverse the circumstances are, all the time. These recipes would not only help you feel better but they are really nutritious too.

You can either make your survival even tougher for you by eating food that is not tasty because you're too busy thinking about survival while you make your food. Or you can go ahead try these recipes that could help you lighten your mood even when you know times are hard. You have to positive. And to be positive, you would have to eat positive. Without being positive, you will not be able to survive as it is an essential thing to do. Best of luck!

Survive a Disaster

Introduction

Have you always wondered what you would do if a disaster has struck down and you have to survive without any help for a long period of time? In this book, you would be reading about surviving the toughest situations and training your mind on how to face fear and use it for your own advantage. You would learn what things you would need to survive in harsh circumstances. I have shared some ideas on storing enough water for your survival until help comes to you. I have discussed the preservation of food in one chapter too. There is a whole chapter about first aid in which I have tried my best to explain how to handle certain injuries and wounds when you have no help.

You cannot survival adverse situations if your mind if fearful. I have explained how you can face your fears and train your mind to be able to survive the scariest of situations. You would also read about basic survival skills needed to survive.

I have explained every strategy and tip in a way that it is easy for everyone to understand. You would also learn to defend yourself against people who, in order to survive, would try to harm you just to get to your supplies.

Disasters and bad times are a part of your lives and you will find this book really helpful in coping with such circumstances.

Chapter 1 - Must Have Survival Skills

There is just so much to learn when it comes to surviving in difficult circumstances. You would not even know where to start learning? I am going to share with you the basic survival skills that everybody should have if he/she wants to survive when the times are hard.

In this chapter, you would learn the 6 basic survival strategies that you need when the times are hard and adverse. Let's have a look at the 6 strategies.

Strategy# 1 - Your Attitude:

The number one strategy is your attitude. Your survival depends mostly on your attitude, how you handle different survival situations. Your attitude would decide if you would live or die. So you have to concentrate on your attitude first.

Let me share with you "The Rule of Threes". The rule is as follows,

- You can survive for 3 minutes without air

- You can only survive 3 hours without a regulated body temperature (a proper shelter)

- You can only live for 3 days without water

- You cannot live for more than 3 weeks without food

This rule also guides you about the important of different things for your survival.

Air>Shelter>Water>Food

Surviving a disaster also requires that you do not panic in the face of survival challenges. When you encounter a survival threat, remember this word, **SPEAR.**

Stop
Plan
Execute
Assess
Re-evaluate

To address a difficult and harsh situation, it is very important that you do everything in a calm manner and systematically. This will keep your body and mind fully focused on the matter at hand and keeps you from panicking or getting all sorts of negative vibes. With a resilient and strong attitude, your chances to survive any threat are greatly enhanced.

Strategy# 2 - Shelter:

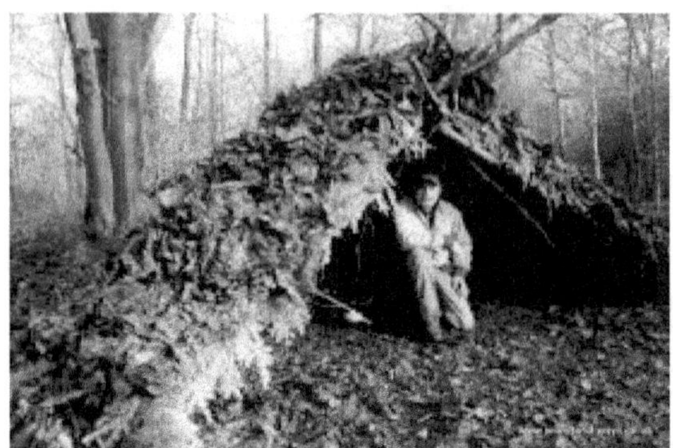

Shelter is very important when you face a survival situation. How? When you are in a survival situation and you don't have a proper shelter, you would be exposed to different elements that may harm your body and make you weak physically and mentally. So you should be able to build a shelter for you to survive any potential harsh condition. It is paramount that you avoid heat loss in your body and in hot circumstances; you have to keep yourself hydrated and prevent water loss in your body to keep you going on. You can build a shelter considering the following points,

- The location should be away from any hazards and near materials that you would need.

- The shelter should be able to insulate you from ground, rain, wind, sun etc.

- The shelter should be near a heat source.

There are many types of natural shelters you can consider when facing a survival threat. You can take shelter in a cave or a hollow stump. Building a shelter with logs is also useful. In cold areas, building a snow hut is very useful. A debris hut is the most practical shelter that you can build to live in the face of potential survival threats.

Strategy# 3 - Water:

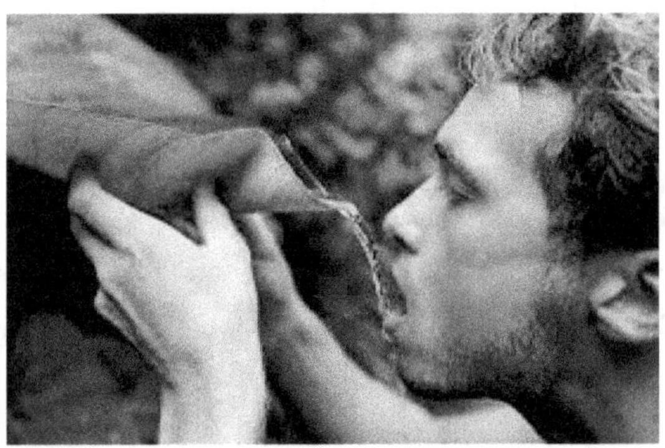

https://encrypted-tbno.gstatic.com/images?q=tbn:ANd9GcQ98W8WmmEtZ7SXDXEg6XoIX-kPmkpHlF6BKJKRUKyqCxTV6Hb2qw

A human body consists mainly of water, up to 78%. This is why water is more important than food or fire. In ideal situations, a person consumes at least a gallon of water daily. People who survive the destruction caused by the disasters, often die because of dehydration or drinking unclean and unhealthy water. Unclean water can have various fatal bacteria, germs and pathogens. In addition to germs and pathogens, many streams and lakes contain industrial and agricultural waste which is also a cause of death because such water contains metals or elements that are seriously harmful for a human body. The best sources of water that are pure and harmless to human body are springs and small water tributaries. You can also collect morning dew which is pure too.

Filtering pumps and chemical treatments like iodine are the most popular ways of cleaning water before drinking it. If you have access to these elements, you would not have to worry about the water problem. There are many natural herbs that can clean water from germs and bacteria. Grapefruit seed extract is a very famous herbal water purifier but, there is still research going on, if it is 100% useful or not. The best way to purify water is to boil it. Cook water until big bubbles start to come to the top. Then keep boiling the water for 2-3 minutes will ensure that all the germs and bacteria are dead.

You can survive for weeks if you have an upright attitude, a good shelter and if you are drinking clean water.

Strategy# 4 - Fire:

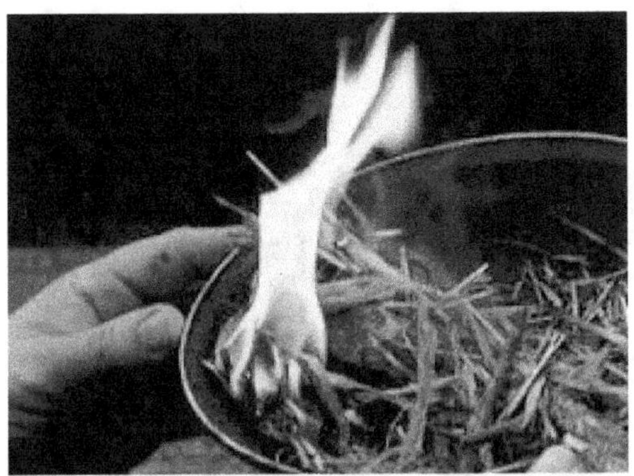

Fire is very important when you are facing a survival situation. It helps keep your body and shelter warm. You can dry your clothes, boil water and cook food for yourself with fires. Fire is also important to give you a sense of security and safety in a survival situation because different wild animals and preys can be scared off by fire.

It is ideal to carry fir starting tools with you almost all the time because who knows when you would be facing a survival condition. Keep a lighter with you, or matches, flint or steel etc. In adverse weather, it would be challenging to start a fire even if you have any of these implements. It is very important that you learn some basic fire-making skills to keep yourself ready if a disaster strikes down and you have to survive difficult times. Starting fire by friction is the most popular way of starting a fire. The most famous fire-making methods are bow drill method, fire plough method and fire saw method etc.

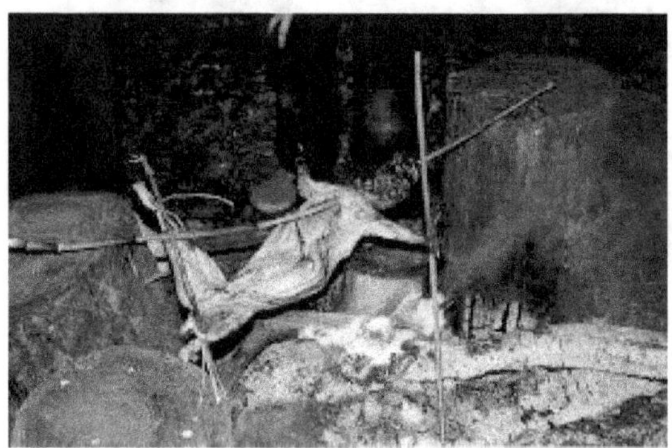

https://encrypted-tbn2.gstatic.com/images?
q=tbn:ANd9GcRwQZj3dICEGanxRNHuyqvFfuC8vPCK6WeJkK_qSsYJ3
WyN9zLZ

This strategy is about being able to identify different plants that you can eat. As compared to water and shelter, you can survive longer without food. You can survive without food for 3 weeks. But you would become weak still. Our environment is full of different eatables if you just know what to eat. Wild plants are a great source of nutritional food but you have to be very careful because there are fruits and berries and herb that are poisonous too. So make sure you know what you are going to what when you are facing a survival challenge.

I have a list of plants that can be a god source of nutritional food for you,

- Cattail – You can eat the roots, shoots and the pollen heads.

- Conifers – You can eat the inner bark which is called the Cambium. It is full of sugars, starches and calories. You can find this on most of the evergreen and cone-bearing trees. Yew is poisonous.

- Grasses – You can drink the juices from the leaves. They are very nutritious. The root corm, you can roast and eat.

- Oaks –Leach the tannic acids from acorns and eat them. Acorns are a good source of fats, proteins and calories for you.

PRECAUTION: Use field guides to identify different roots, herbs and plants because there are many plants that are eatable but they have poisonous identical too that are exactly the same. So if you are not sure about a plant, don't eat it.

Strategy# 6 - Naturalistic Knowledge:

The sixth skill that you need to survive a natural disaster is to have naturalistic knowledge. The more you know about nature, the more chances are of your survival. If you have wildlife tracking skills, it would be easy for you to catch game for your food and hunt. If you know different herbs and plants, it would be easy for you to find the right food to eat and use different herbs to treat different illnesses and injuries. Having a good knowledge about your body and how different organs are inter-related can help a lot in a survival situation. You would be able to utilize your resources in a more useful manner.

You should have a basic knowledge about natural sciences too like Botany, Geology, Zoology, Ecology etc.

The 6 strategies that I have discussed in this chapter are the most important things for your survival. If you can take care of these 6 points, you would be able to survive longer than anybody else.

Chapter 2 - Learn First Aid to Handle Injuries

In this chapter, I have given the next 2 important tips and strategies need for survival.

Strategy# 7 - Knowing different injuries and wounds and how to take care of them

Strategy# 8 - Medications to keep with you to treat different injuries

In a survival situation, you will not have access to hospitals or medicines. Your best hope would be your own self. Which means you should be able to provide first aid to yourself and to others if need be. I have explained here about different basic injuries and wounds and how you can recognize them and treat them.

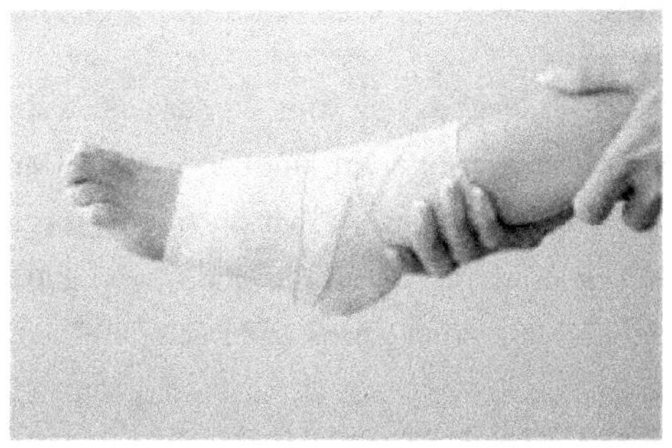

https://encrypted-tbn3.gstatic.com/images?q=tbn:ANd9GcQYwVqrSrAUnO8kYpLKXhGWkbASGg9k9X31hTEyXsk7zPo6GPFdDQ

What is an injury?

Any damage to your body is an injury. These are caused by accidents, hits, falls, bites, cuts, weapons etc. Injuries can be minor as well as fatal.

Here is a list of different kinds of injuries and how you can take care of them,

- Wounds

- Bruises

- Burns

- Dislocations

- Sprains and strains

Wounds - When an injury opens up your skin or your body tissues, it's called a wound. Cuts, scrapes etc are different kinds of wounds. Minor wounds are not serious but you have to clean them so that they don't get infected. You can use clean water to first clean all the blood from the wound and then you can use an antiseptic to keep it from getting germs and bacteria. Then you can cover it up with a clean bandage or piece of cloth. Deeper wounds need to be stitched. To be able to do that you should get first-aid lessons.

Bruises - It is also called a contusion or Ecchymoses. A bruise is an injury that happens when your blood is trapped under your skin. It happens when the impact cruses the blood vessel but the skin doesn't open up to get the blood out. So the blood gets trapped under your skin when it doesn't find a way to get out.

Such injuries are painful and the effected part might get swollen. You can get bruises on your skin, you muscles or even your bones. Bone bruises are the most serious ones.

How to treat bruises?

Bruises are reddish in colour and they turn purple or greenish before they heal. Bruises take months to heal but you can reduce the effect by applying ice on the affected area and lifting the part above your heart.

Burns – Burns are caused by the exposure of heat, chemicals or radiations to your body. Burns damage your skin and body tissues. Internal burns are also caused when you inhale in smoke or flammable gasses.

Burns are of three types,

- First-degree burns are when only the outer skin is damaged.

- Second-degree burns are when the next layer of your outer skin is damaged too.

- Third-degree burns are when the damage is too deep and the tissues are burnt too.

How to treat burns?

In case of minor burns, make sure the burned are doesn't get infected. Clean the injury and apply antibiotic creams on the area. Burns are very much prone to getting infected because the protective barrier of your skin is broken. So make sure the wound is clean and covered. Apply calamine lotion on the burnt area.

Dislocations - It is when the ends of your bones are dislocated. This happens as a result of a fall or a blow. When your bones are dislocated, it is visible and the area is usually swollen. You won't be able to move the dislocated part.

The best way to locate the bone back to the normal position is to do just push it back to the right place. This requires learning how to do it. After the dislocated joint has been returned to normal position, use a splint or a sling to keep it there and let the bones heal for a few days or weeks.

Sprains and Strains – These can happen as a result of falling, twisting or getting hit. A sprain happened when ligaments are stretched or torn. Ligaments are the tissues that are a connection between bones and the joint. The part will swell up and get bruised.

When a muscle or tendon is torn or stretched, it's called strain. Tendons are tissues that tear if you twist or pull your body part too hard, the muscles would swell and cause pain and you would get muscles spasms too as a result of a strain.

How to treat sprains and strains?

To treat sprains and strains, you should ice the area and wear a bandage or something that would compress the area. Later when the effects of the sprain or strain are fading, you can start doing minor exercises.

What do you need to treat different injuries?

You should also know what you would need to treat different sorts of injuries with. This is a proven effective tip as you would be keeping medication that would help you survive different injuries and wounds. You should keep the following medications with you,

- Antibiotic ointment - To prevent minor wounds or injuries from getting infected

- Hydrocortisone cream - To reduce chemical reactions on the skin

- Calamine lotion - To relieve pain and prevent itching caused by poison, insect bites, burns or rashes

- Antihistamine, such as diphenhydramine - For allergic reactions

- Antiseptic solution or ointment - To clean wounds or injuries

- Aloe Vera gel - to heal wounds or skin inflammation

Chapter 03 - Tips for Storage of Water and Food

In the face of adverse circumstances, it is important that you have enough food and water stored to keep you going for a long period of time. In this chapter I would share two more effective strategies with you,

Strategy# 9 - How to store water?

As water is more important to human life than food, let's discuss that first.

How much water do I need?

In ideas conditions, a single person consumes a gallon of water every day. Half a gallon is used for drinking purposes and the other half is used for hygiene.

How much water should you store for your survival?

According to experts, you should always have water you can consume for 3 days because after that you are likely to get help. But if some huge disaster strikes down, it's possible that you might not get aid for weeks and even month. So it is recommended that you store water that you can use in 2 weeks. This is just a start up. You can start by saving 2 weeks' worth water and then add up with time and money.

How can you store water for long periods of time?

If you are planning on storing water for long periods of time, you have to find a safe container to store the water in. You can use plastic bottles for storing water. Glass bottles are also good for storing water. You can store water in steel containers too but you would not be able to purify the water with Chlorine because the chemical will react with steel and cause rusting. Whatever container that you choose, make sure you can seal the container to prevent the water from harmful bacteria, germs and different dangerous pathogens that contaminate the water!

Water Barrels:

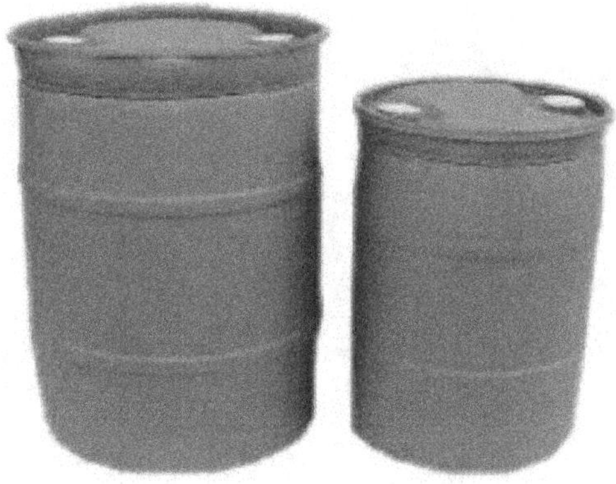

https://encrypted-tbn1.gstatic.com/images?q=tbn:ANd9GcSvI4-RRaBVhsZZL5Z0_7_gqozTzXOk5lDJO2C3sk7F088c1zI3

To store water for longer periods of time, you would need to get 55-gallon water barrels. They are made of food-grade plastic and you can seal them super tight too to keep the water from getting contaminated. These barrels are BPA-free and can keep the water or anything inside them safe from the UV radiations.

To keep these barrels, you would need a lot of space. These barrels are pretty expensive. One barrel can cost you up to $90. Also to fill them up, you would need a pump and a specialty drinking water hose. Also, these barrels and heavy and big and hence, not portable. One full barrel is 440 lbs.

Rain Barrels:

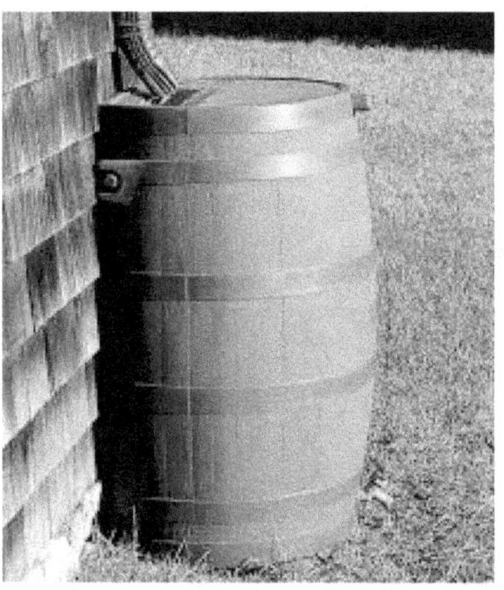

To take advantage of the rain water, you can buy rain barrels too. They are eco-friendly and they don't cost a lot too. All you have to do is to put the rain barrel under the gutter pipe whenever it rains. The barrel would collect the rain water for you. You can store this water. But before you drink it, make sure you sanitize the water and purify it from all the germs and bacteria. You can use the rain water for hygiene and use the water in the water barrels for drinking purposes.

Also I have heard that there are some states that require you to get a permit before you start collecting rain water. And they would even charge you tax for that. Make sure you have checked all the information before you go ahead and start collecting rainwater. You don't want to do anything illegal, do you?

Now that you know how you can store water for prepping, the next effective strategy is about storing food.

Strategy# 10 - How to preserve and store food?

How can I store food?

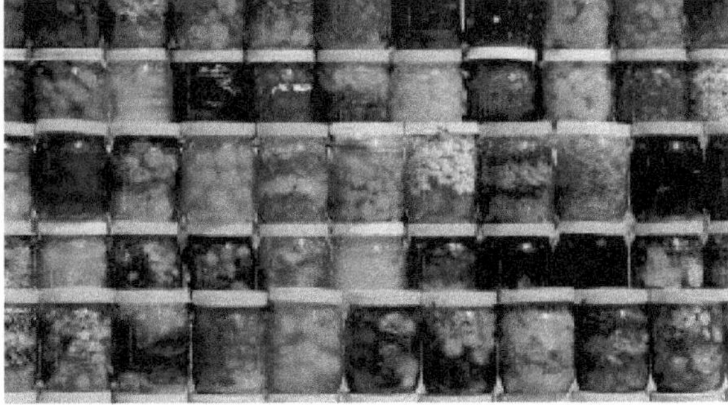

There are many ways through which you can store and preserve food to prep for any disasters. You can store and preserve food for long periods of time by the following ways,

1. **Drying:**

   Drying is the easiest way if preserving food for long. This food preservation method doesn't require a lot of effort. Dry food items and store them for long period of time. As you know, mold grows in wet thing and moisture is vital for its growth so if you are using this method for the preservation of food, you can rest assured that your food is free from any bacteria and germs. Your dried food would stay for long without rotting or catching germs.

2. **Canning:**

   Canning is one of the traditional ways to preserve food. You can your food by cooking it partially so that all the bacteria and germs are dead. Then you can add certain additives like sugar syrup etc. After this you can clean the jars, dry them and put the partially cooked food items in the jars and seal them tight. You can keep these jars stored somewhere for a long time.

3. **Salt curing:**

   Salt curing is an old method by which you can preserve meat for a long time. Salt is used to keep the meat safe from bacteria because germs

cannot survive in an environment where there is more than 10% of salt
concentration. Meat is rubbed with a mixture of salt and sugar and then it
is put in a jar or a pot that is shut super tight and kept where the
temperature is cool

4. Refrigeration:

This is the most common way of preservation of food. You can keep cooked
food and raw meat in the refrigerator to keep them safe for a long period of
time. And when you need to eat the food, you can defrost it and cook it.

If you are able to keep enough food and water for your survival in the times of
disasters, you would not have to worry about these basic human needs and you
would be able to concentrate on other problems that you might face during harsh
situations.

Chapter 04 - Train Your Mind for Survival Mentality

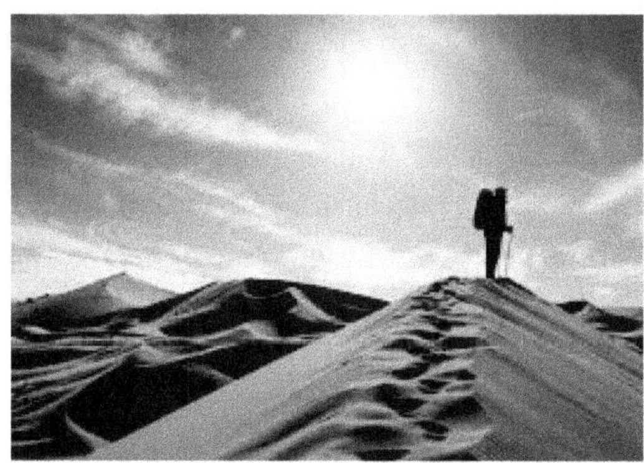

The most important thing you need for survival is a calm and brave mind. If your mind is panicking and you cannot concentrate on surviving, you might not live long. In this chapter, I would give you 5 tips on how you can make a mind that will get you through all the adverse circumstances. But first there are a few things that I would like to discuss.

What is survival?

To be prepared to survive, to control your fears, to take control of your emotions, keep your ego in check. This is what survival is all about. It's not just about food, water and shelter. You have to have a sound mind and the ability to survive to actually survive a disaster.

Now, if you have knowledge about herbs, plants, how to make a fire, how to make a small hut etc, it would not be enough to keep you alive if you don't have the survival mentality. You have to be able to think clearly and make decisions fast to keep living in adverse circumstances.

If your mind is not strong enough, no amount of prepping would help you survive when a disaster strikes down.

How do you survive?

The answer to this is your mentality, how your mind confronts adverse situations. Survivors don't accept that they are helpless, they don't accept death even if they are so close to it. They have a **will to survive.** They refuse to let the circumstances decide if they would live or not. They choose to survive no matter what.

Without the **will to survive,** not even the most trained survivors would stand a chance against the circumstances. Knowing what you need to survive is very important but having a **will to survive** is the most important thing you need to survive.

A mindset that doesn't surrender and wants to live is the key to your survival in the most difficult circumstances.

Effects of fear on your mind:

There are two ways in which fear affects different people's mind,

1. Some people let the fear take over their mind. So much that they are unable to make any decisions on how to survive the situation. They are so scared that their ability to decide stops working. They close their eyes and give themselves to the fear and this kind of mindset leads them to their downfall.

2. There are people that use their fear to make quick decisions in order to rid themselves of the situation that is causing all the fear. These people allow their adrenaline to take over and this leads to hasty decisions. Because they don't get a chance to think clearly, they make wrong decisions and instead of solving the problem, create more problems for themselves.

Survival Mindset:

To survive in the most stressful circumstances, it is important that you control the flow of your thoughts, think calmly, don't panic and control your anxiety and your fears. Take control of your mind and be the master of yourself. If you let your mind control you, you would not survive. If you have a survival mindset and you can take a situation into your hands without panicking, you would be able to do things you never thought you could.

The last five tips on how to survive the most difficult of circumstances are probably the most important of all the tips that I have given you in this book. These tips include,

Strategy# 11 - Control your fear:

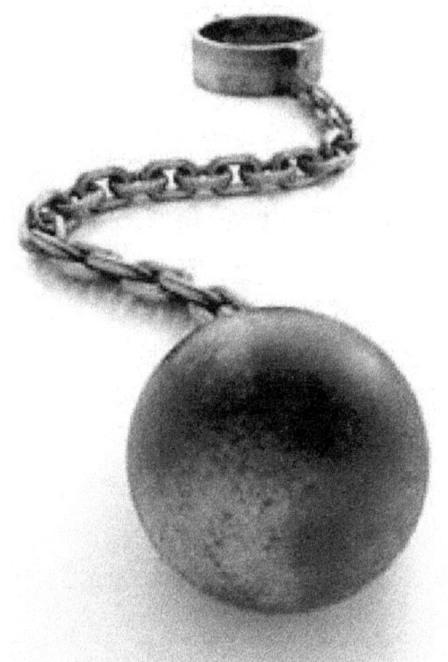

https://encrypted-tbn3.gstatic.com/images?q=tbn:ANd9GcQLMLvAcry1T_D1WGIRctFHl4DlCKcLQP-ffpqXhPdC6YjGnYp-

You have to control your fears and not panic. This is the first thing you should be able to do. When you face a life or death situation, you have to control your fear of ending up dead, because this very fear would get you killed. Just keep positive thoughts in your mind. Stop and breathe. Calm your mind. Clear your mind of all the negative thoughts and then start analyzing the situation and how you can handle it. You have to keep calm in the face of opposing circumstances, because panicking would only make things worse for you.

Strategy# 12 - Take control of your ego:

Don't panic and don't fear but don't overdo it. Drop that "nothing bad can happen to me" attitude of yours, because it can happen to you. Don't pretend that you have no fears and you can encounter anything without any hesitation or anxiety. That over-confidence can lead to your downfall. You have to be modest. Try to analyze your fears and train yourself in those areas until you are able to control them. Your ego can create bigger problems for you. So it is very important that you control your ego.

Strategy# 13 - Think of positive things:

To be able to think positively even in the face of extremely negative circumstances can lead to your victory. Develop a mindset that is all about positivity. Even if you are in a life or death situation, don't surrender to it. Just think positively and how you can survive the situation.

Strategy# 14 - Do not give in to your fears:

It is very important that you don't surrender to your fears, that you don't close your eyes when the situation is really, really difficult to cope with. The best way to survive any situation is to digest your fears, and try your best to fight the difficult situation. If you give in to your fears, you would end up dead.

Strategy# 15 - Keep training:

The last tip to survive any disaster is to be prepared all the time. Keep training yourself for the worst of circumstances. You can train yourself by practicing basic survival skills. Even if the circumstances are well and good, be prepared for the worst. The key to surviving sudden natural disasters is to be prepared all the time because who knows when a disaster strikes down.

Conclusion

To survive in the harshest of circumstances, one needs to be always prepared. You can do so by reading this book and understand everything. You can start practicing because disasters don't announce before they come. So if the circumstances become adverse suddenly, you have to be prepared for them beforehand.

You have to prep for different kinds of situations. In this book, you have learnt how you can tackle different survival situations. You have to store and preserve enough food to be able to survive times when you have no access to food. Human life cannot go on without water. You have to keep a considerable amount of water to keep you going until the circumstances are back to normal.

I hope that we never have to face circumstances that require these survival strategies and tips, but if we do, we would be prepared to face them. One thing that is really, really important is your mind set and your attitude in the face of adverse conditions. If you give in to the bad situations, it would be the death of you. If you want to live, you have to prepare a mind that is free from anxiety and that doesn't panic in the most panicky situations. **The Will to Survive** is the main key to surviving even the most difficult of situations. Good luck!

Survival Medicine

Introduction

Accidents can happen anytime without former notice. This means you need to be prepared beforehand for emergency situations. Standing by an accident and not being able to do anything to help makes things more unpleasant. For such cases, you should be ready to give prompt and basic aid to the sufferer/s until the professionals jump in and take care of the situation. First aid is important because it helps controlling an emergency situation so that it doesn't get out of hand.

You should always have a first-aid kit with you and a medical handbook that has basic medical guidelines for you. In this book, you'll know what you need to do to make a complete first-aid kit that has everything you need in a survival situation or if you happen to witness an accident.

Time is very important in case of emergency situations. A person can literally die within seconds if he/she is not given basic medical attention. In this book, I'd teach you how to avoid that, how to save someone's life without losing a second.

For this book to help you fully, you'd need a lot of courage. Emergencies and accidents are not for the faint-hearted people. The sight of blood, suffering, injuries and even simple wounds can shake you if you are not brave enough. So first of all, you'd have to be brave for someone else so that he/she can be saved. It'd not be difficult if you really think about the difference you'd be making in somebody else's life. You could be saving lives so stand up and be brave for humanity.

This book would help you understand why first-aid is important and how can you set up your own first aid kit that has everything you need for every possible emergency.

Chapter 1 – Why is Survival Medicine Important for You?

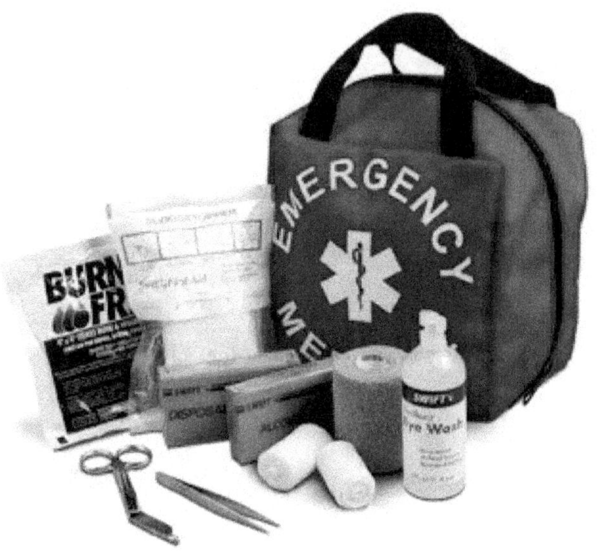

First things first! Why is survival medicine important when you have doctors and paramedics to help? The answer is simple. Suppose you're driving back home and on your way back you witness two cars colliding each other. What would you do? You'd stop your car and you'll call 911 in an instant. Now, it's obvious that it would take time for 911 to reach the site of an accident. What would you do until then? Wait? No, because, there are a bunch of people bleeding immensely. They might be in a critical condition situation. Now waiting for the professionals to come and handle the situation that is getting worse with every passing second, would not be a wise decision on your end. How would you feel if you had a first aid kit and knowledge of survival medicine to help you alleviate the suffering of the people in distress? This is why survival medicine is really important, for situations like these.

Survival medicine is important because only then you'd be able to give initial assistance to someone who's injured or ill. Initial assistant is just to control a deteriorating situation so that it doesn't get out of hand until the professionals arrive. First-aid can be given by a layperson with some basic equipment and medicine in their first-aid kit. And if you don't have that, you'd just be a bystander who'd see the situation getting worse and would not be able to do anything about it.

Benefits of Survival Medicine and Quick Medical Assistance

Let's have a look at some of the benefits of survival medicine and quick medical assistance,

- **Your family and home would be safe:** The biggest benefit of learning first aid and quick medical assistance is that your home would be a safe place. How? You'd be more and more cautious about things and if there's an accident, you'd be able to take things under your control and alleviate your family member's suffering until the doctors reach you.

- **Your workplace would be safer:** You know how to give quick medical assistance in times of need; this means your workplace would feel a lot safer with you. If your colleague is having a seizure or is physically hurt somehow, you'd be able to help him/her.

- **You can save lives:** If you know how to give instant medical assistance to a person in distress, you are a life saver. You can save a lot of lives if a natural disaster strikes down or if there's a road accident on your way home.

- **It can reduce recovery time:** Wounds and injuries take a lot of time to heal if they're left open and unattended for a long period of time and this is very common when someone is injured in a road accident and the paramedics are on their way. If you are there at the time of a road accident and you know how to stop the wound from getting infected and you have a first-aid medical of your own too, it would help reduce the recovery time of the wound or injury.

- **You could help the suffering person in an emergency or distress:** If you're there when a person suddenly gets an asthma attack, or swallows something poisonous, or gets ill or if a natural disaster occurs, you'd not just be a bystander like most of the people standing there. You'd be able to help not only the suffering party but you'd also be able to stop things from getting worse even for the paramedics and doctors.

- **You could assist the suffering party in the right way:** This is very important that the person suffering gets the right treatment. If you're not knowledgeable about how to give the right medical assistance to the person suffering, you might make things worse to an extent that the even professionals won't be able to handle it. Survival medicine in first-aid ensures that you know exactly what you're doing and you're confident about it.

- **You could help yourself:** Your first-aid and survival medicine knowledge is not just helpful to other people in distress; you could also make use of this knowledge to help yourself too.

Accidents keep happening and we don't know when or where we would have to face an emergency situation. To be able to tackle situations like these, it is important that you have first-aid knowledge. Fatalities often are a result of lack of instant medical treatment. Survival medicine and first-aid would ensure that quick medical assistance is given to not only stop the matters from getting out of our hands but also to save lives. And keeping a first-aid kit and a medical handbook with you always would help you tackle sudden emergencies.

Chapter 2 – Setting Up Your First-Aid Kit

Knowledge of survival medicine and first-aid alone is of no use if you don't have the necessary equipment and medicines to help you carry out the required treatments. For example, if you find an injured person bleeding out on the road and you know how to take care of his wounds and how to bandage him, what medicines to use but you don't have those medicines with you and it would take some time until help arrives and there's no pharmacy nearby either. What good would your knowledge of survival medicine be if you can't help someone in distress? For cases such as these, what you need is a first-aid kit with you.

Carrying a well-equipped first-aid kit with you all the time would help you cope with sudden natural disasters, road-side accidents, sudden illness, injuries and wounds etc. There are many drugstores and pharmacies where you could get your hands on a good first-aid kit. But I suggest that you assemble a first-aid kit of your own. In this chapter, you'd know what necessary medicines and equipment you should have to complete your own first-aid kit.

Here's a list of supplies and medicines and other necessary stuff that are essential for a complete and well-stocked first-aid kit.

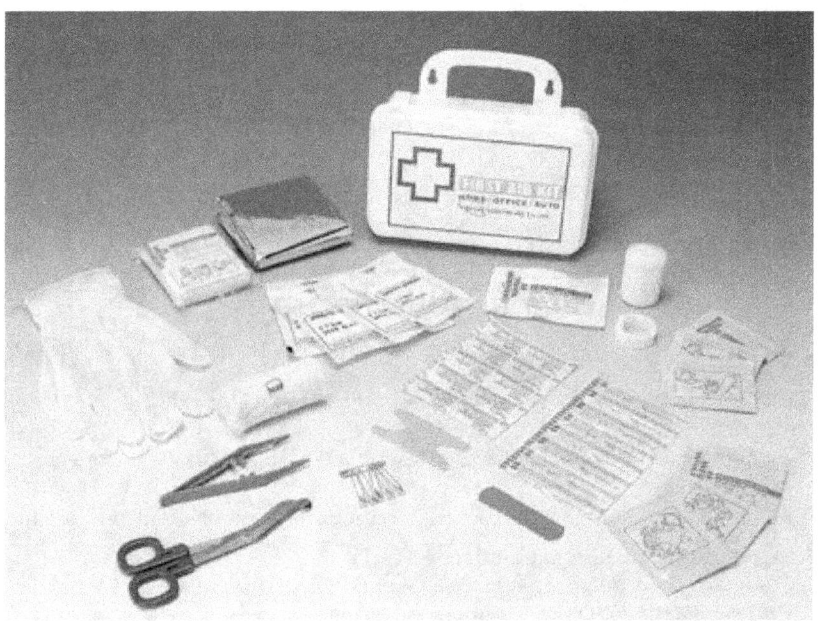

Basic Supplies You Need in Your First-Aid Kit

First, you'd need to get some basic supplies for your first-aid kit. Here's a list of these supplies,

- A water bottle - To drink or clean wounds or injuries

- Disposable non-latex examination gloves, several pairs - To prevent bacteria and germs from hands to transfer to a wound or injury

- Adhesive tape - To hold splints or dressing together

- Duct tape

- Cotton balls and cotton buds - To apply ointments or other solutions to wounds or injuries

- Absorbent cotton rolls - To use as a padding for a splint

- Eye pads

- Elastic wrap bandages

- Bandage strips (Different sizes) - To use on minor or major cuts and abrasions

- Butterfly bandages - To hold the cuts together to let them heal

- Roller gauzes (Different sizes) - To support sprained muscles or sore parts

- Sterile gauze pads - To control bleeding or secretions and prevent the injury or wound from festering

- Triangular bandages - To support a broken limb

- A lubricant (Petroleum jelly)

- Aluminum finger splint

- Instant cold packs - For contusions or bruises

- Plastic bags (Different sizes)

- Safety pins (Different sizes)

- Scissors

- Tweezers

- Hand sanitizer - To keep your hands germs and bacteria free

- Thermometer

- Suction device (Turkey baster)

- Breathing barrier

- Syringes

- Medicine cups or spoons

- Face and dust masks - To protect against dust, germs or allergens

- A First-aid manual

Next, you'd need to get the following medications for your first-aid kit,

- Eyewash solution

- Antibiotic ointment - To prevent minor wounds or injuries from getting infected

- Calamine lotion - To relieve pain and prevent itching caused by poison, insect bites, burns or rashes

- Antacids - To reduce symptoms of Acid Reflux

- Antiseptic solution or ointment - To clean wounds or injuries

- Aloe vera gel - to heal wounds or skin inflammation

- Anti-diarrhea medication

- Laxative - To increase bowel movements

- Antihistamine, such as diphenhydramine - For allergic reactions

- Pain relievers, (Tylenol, Advil, Ibuprofen, Aspirins etc) - Aspirin is not for children

- Hydrocortisone cream - To reduce chemical reactions on the skin

- Cough and cold medications

In the case of emergencies, you should be all set. Below is a list of items you would need in emergencies,

- A list of emergency phone numbers like emergency road service providers, poison helpline etc

- A small flashlight that is water resistant

- Extra batteries

- Waterproof writing equipment and notepads

- Waterproof matches

- A phone with a solar charger

- Insect repellents

- Sunscreen

The lists given above contain everything that you would need in times of emergencies. If you get everything from the list, you'd be able to handle any problem you come across.

Some Precautions

Now that you have all that you need in your first-aid kit, here are some of the precautions you have to make sure that you'd take care of,

- Keep your first-aid kit away from the reach of your children.

- Always take your first-aid kit with you, wherever you go. Even to work.

- Always read the instructions on the medication before you take them.

- Keep a special check on the expiry dates of the medications you have in your first-aid kit. Make sure you've disposed of the medicines that have expired and replaced them with fresh ones.

- Aspirins are not for children. Don't give it to them.

- Don't buy medicines that have cuts or tears on their packs.

- Make sure you know all about the medicines you have in your first-aid kit.

- Consider participating in a first-aid course provided by different organizations.

- Teach your children a little about first-aid too, depending on their age.

If you have everything mentioned in this chapter, fear not, you'd be able to cope almost all sorts of emergency situations that require instant medical attention. Keep this first-aid kit with you everywhere you go and prove yourself useful to the people in distress.

Chapter 3 – Maintain Your First-Aid Kit

You've completed your medical first aid-kit. It's good news that you've not gotten any chance to use it because that means, you have not encountered an emergency or a natural disaster or a road accident etc. But it doesn't mean you can leave your first-aid kid unattended. Once you've set up your first-aid kit, it doesn't mean, your job has finished and that this was all to it. No. It's a continuous job. You cannot just leave your first-aid kit in some corner of your room. You'd have to keep a check on it. You'd have to see if the medications have expired. If yes, you'd have to dispose of them immediately. It is a very common mistake that we make with everything. We buy something and we think that this is it and there's nothing more you should do. That's not true. Let's say, for example, you've bought a car, would leave it like that in the garage forever even if you're using it regularly? No. you won't, because, that way it would stop working eventually. Why? Because, you have done nothing to take care of it! You have never checked if your car needed maintenance. Yes! Just like your car and everything else, you'd need to maintain your first-aid kit too. Here's how you can do that.

How to maintain your first-aid kit?

After you've gotten all the supplies and medications for your first-aid kit, you'd need to store them in some place safe and where they are not open to getting contaminated. This is very important that you make sure your first-aid kit is somewhere, 1) Safe and clean and 2) you can access it anytime you want.

Some tips on maintaining your first-aid kit,

- **Select the right container:** This is the first thing you should be doing. Selecting the right container for your supplies and medicines. Get a container that is water resistant. This is important because it can happen that you have to work in the rain. Select a container that is lightweight and durable. There are many options in the market that you can choose from.

- **Keep the supplies in an order:** To maintain your first-aid kit as efficiently as possible, you'd have to make sure you do that in an orderly manner. Whether your first-aid kit is a box or a bag, you should make sure that everything is kept in an orderly fashion. Why? Because there are certain liquids and solutions that can spill in your kit damaging other supplies too which means you'd not be able to use almost anything from your first-aid kit. So order is the first step to maintaining your first-aid kit.

- **Keep the liquids and fluids tight shut -** To avoid any spills, you have to make sure all the solutions and liquids in your first-aid kit are tightly shut. You don't have to be an expert to understand that liquid spill can damage other supplies too. And then you'd have to unpack and repack your whole first-aid medical kit again.

- **Keep your first-aid medical kit at room temperature -** Wherever you want to keep your first-aid kit, make sure the temperature is not very high and not very low. Because there are medicines in your first-aid kit that require to be kept at room temperature to keep them from damaging.

Keep your first-aid medical kit organized

Why do you want to do this? Because there are just so many things stuffed in your first-aid kid that in times of need, you might want something, let's say you want the bandages. Where are the bandages? They might be somewhere beneath all the pile of other bandages, cotton balls and gauzes. A lot of time would be wasted in finding just the bandages. What would happen when you'd need to find other tablets and medications? To save time and lives, it is mighty important that you keep your first-aid kit in an organized way. How can you do that? You can divide all the supplies and medicines into a few categories. The categories can be,

1. Equipment to treat wounds and injuries

2. Prescription medication

3. Ointments and solutions

4. Other supplies

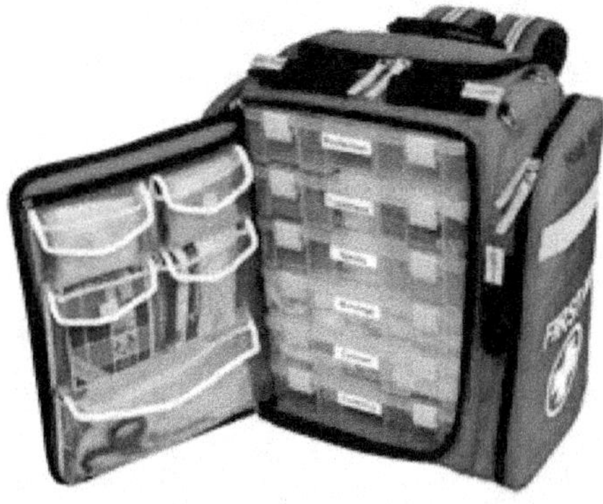

Now keeping in mind these categories, you'd separate all the stuff in four parts. And then you can keep them together in separate sections of your first-aid kit. This way you'd be able to find the right thing in the right section without wasting any time in finding that thing.

Keep updating your first-aid kit

Now that your first-aid kit is all set and you know how to keep it maintained and you are ready to serve humanity in the times of natural disasters or accidents or any such emergencies. But your work doesn't stop here. Like I've said before, your medical kit would need to be checked every now and then. You wouldn't want to end up using expired medication by mistake on the suffering party and make things much, much worse.

Now this is the thing I'll put a lot of emphasis on. This is very important that you keep checking your first-aid kit if it needs anything new, if the medicines and other supplies can still be used or have they expired? Check your kit for any used up supplies. Do that often if you need to use your first-aid kit very often.

It would be really helpful if you keep a checklist of all the items in your first-aid kit with your all the time. With this, you can keep a track of everything that is used up or expired or need replacing. If you don't know what you're doing, it would be really difficult for you to maintain your first-aid kit. But if you do it systematically and in an orderly fasion, one thing at a time, it would be really easy.

Yes. It is true that keeping a first-aid medical kit is not a fun job but nobody does it for fun. It's done to serve humanity and help people out when they need it. Keeping a first-aid medical kit can cost you a lot. It doesn't matter if you've bought a ready-made first-aid medical kit or you've built yourself one, it is always going to cost you. You'd always have to keep checking it and buy new supplies that have either expired or finished up. But this shouldn't stop you from getting a first-aid medical kit because this is something that you don't do for money but for the sake of a good cause. Plus, if ever you need to use your first-aid medical kit, you'd realize that it was worth every penny that you've spent setting it up and maintaining it.

Chapter 4 – Necessary Things You Need in Your Medical Handbook

In the previous chapters you have learned how to set up a first-aid medical kit for yourself and how to maintain that medical kit in order to keep it working for you. Now that you have learnt how to set up a first-aid medical kit and how to take care of it in the best way possible, what should you need more to be able to do everything there is to help the suffering party? A complete medical handbook of course!

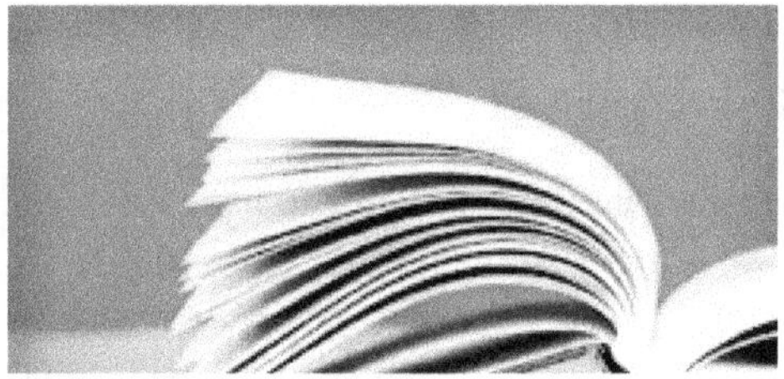

Why do you need a medical handbook?

The answer to this question is really simple. If you face an emergency situation that you have no knowledge about, a medical handbook would help you handle it. A medical handbook would teach you simple procedures like how to cover a wound and prevent it from getting infected, or how to give a CPR, or how to handle deep cuts and wounds etc.

Now the question that next comes to mind is what kind of a medical handbook should you keep with you always? Obviously, there are many medical handbooks available in the market that cover all kinds of medical topics. Which one should you choose for your guidance? Below are some points that you should keep in mind before you buy a medical handbook to keep with your first-aid kit.

- Buy a basic book that some basic stuff about quick medical treatment and first-aid.

- Don't buy a book that has a lot of pro stuff written in it.

- Look for a medical handbook that has step by step guidelines as well as pictures to explain different medical treatments and situations to you.

- Buy a book that is easy to understand. A book that a layperson can keep for his/her guidance.

- Buy a book that would teach you how to handle emergency situations in simple and easy steps.

- This handbook should contain guidelines about simple quick medical treatments like CPR, stroke treatment etc.

About what medical emergencies should my medical handbook offer me guidelines?

The answer to this question is a difficult one because there are so many different medical situations that you may have to face all of a sudden and to say how can you be prepared for all of them, would not be rational. But there are some general and main medical assistance procedures that come on handy in almost all kinds of emergencies. Be it a natural disaster or a road accident or an animal bite. Let's dig deeply into the above points and see what treatments and medical guidelines your medical handbook should offer you that can prove helpful in almost all emergency situations.

- **Short breathing** - Your medical handbook should be able to guide you on how to cope with a situation in which the victim is having difficulties breathing.

- **Choking** - Your medical handbook should guide you on how to help someone who's choking. The handbook should explain the symptoms of choking and how to treat it.

- **Nosebleed** - This is is a common medical situation. Your medical handbook should be able to guide you on causes of nosebleed and how to treat them instantly.

- **Broken bones** - Before you get the victim to a doctor or a doctor comes to him/her, you should be able to give some quick medical assistance to the suffering person so that matters don't get out of your hands by the time the doctor arrives. This should all be explained in easy term in your medical handbook.

- **Avoid infections** - Injuries and wounds are really sensitive areas. They are a way for the bacterias and germs to get into the body easily. If they remain open for a long period of time and are not cleaned up, they may get infected which would make the matters worse than they were before. Your medical handbook should guide you on how to clean minor or major wounds and how to prevent them from getting infected.

- **Bruises and contusions** - Bruises and contusions are common and they must be taken care of. Your medical handbook should tell you how to treat different bruises and contusions on a human body.

- **Alleviate pain** - When the sufferer is in pain, you'd first need to lessen his suffering by giving him pain relievers. There should be enough information on the use and dose of pain killers in your medical handbook.

- **Treat allergies** - Your medical handbook should explain how to treat different kinds of allergies and the causes behind them.

- **Treat bites, poisons and stings** - Getting bit by a stray dog, or a snake or a wasp's sting is something not very rare. Your medical handbook should tell you how to treat different bites and stings before you take the victim to the doctor.

- **Heat stroke -** This is something that is common in places that are hot and humid. Your medical handbook should contain information and guidelines on how to treat heat stroke.

- **Vomiting and nausea -** Get a medical handbook that has guidelines about treating vomiting and nausea in case of emergencies.

- **Seizures -** A complete medical handbook should teach the reader on how to handle a person who is having different kinds of seizures. How to help him until the professionals arrive.

- **High fever -** If someone's suffering from a high fever, you should have a medical handbook that has guidelines on how to keep the fever from going up and maintain body temperature until the doctors come to the rescue.

- **Frostnip -** It is a mild freezing cold wound and your medical handbook should have information on the symptoms and how to treat it.

- **Frostbite -** Make sure that you've bought a handbook that can teach you how to treat frostbite and what are the causes and the symptoms.

- **Hypothermia -** Temperature drops and severe cold can cause the human body to lose its temperature. Make sure that you have selected a medical handbook that has enough information on how to identify the symptoms of hypothermia and how to treat it.

- **Gas inhalation -** If someone's inhaled a dangerous gas, you should know what to do about it. Buy a medical handbook that can help you recognize what kind of gas the victim has inhaled and how it can be treated.

- **Use of basic medical equipment in your first-aid kit -** Your medical handbook should cover all there is about different basic medical equipment that one keeps in a first-aid box.

This was a more specific list of things you should have in your medical handbook that you've bought. Make sure your medical handbook provides assistance to the above problems because they are the most common problems you'll be facing in the times of distress. You'd need the medical handbook to help you when you're confused and not sure about what to do with a certain kind of problem. Finding the best medical handbook that would help you handle almost all kinds of emergency situations is not an easy job. So take your time and deeply search for the best medical handbook out there. Don't make haste. Scan and skim through different medical handbooks before you finally decide on buying the right one. Because you don't want to face an emergency and realize that there is nothing about it in the medical handbook that you have selected. The above list should help you and if you think of anything else that should also be on this list, be open to look for that in your medical handbook too. Otherwise, the above list covers almost everything you'd want in a complete medical handbook.

Conclusion

To conclude this book, I'll say that everyone should set up a first-aid kit and get a medical handbook that contains everything there is to quick medical assistance and first-air. If you've read this book and understood everything, you'd know that first-aid knowledge is really important in times of distress. You could be saving lives and alleviating pain. It's a big task for a layperson.

The best thing about first-aid is that you don't have to be a professional to do this. All you need is some basic medical knowledge (take a first-aid course) and the desire to help humanity to do that if you really wants to do something and make a difference.

With a first-aid kit of your own, you'd not look at other people doe help and you'd certainly not be a helpless spectator or a sad bystander at the site of an emergency or when a natural catastrophe struck down. You'd be someone who could save the day, a superhero, and a person who helped saved lives, someone who really matters.

If you're going to get started with your first-aid kit, good luck. Make sure you have everything in your box and that you take it with you everywhere you go for as I've mentioned earlier, what good would your first-aid kit be if you forget it at home and don't have it when you need it on the road or a trip to some other city.

Also be cautious about maintaining your first-aid kit, keeping in check the expiry dates of all the medications and ointments and different medical solutions. Make sure you buy medicines, bandages, cotton buds etc that have used up. Make a list of all the equipment of your first-aid kit and keep a check on everything that you need to buy because either it's used up or has expired. Because you'd not want to feel helpless if you need a certain medication in an emergency situation but when you check the bottle, it's empty.

Keep the kit safe and away from the reach of your children and make sure it has everything you need, especially when you're leaving your home. Keep it with you every time you leave home. Good luck serving humanity!

Survival Medicine Handbook

Introduction

While the need for medical attention or survival gear can arise in nearly any circumstance, most situations can be treated with the same basic tools and preparations prior to the arrival of medical personnel. With some simple planning, you can stock your kit or pack for just about any circumstance.

A basic emergency kit should not only stock ointments at band aids, but it should include a few tools and items that you may need if you find yourself stranded or away from help. This includes everything from coverage to prevent being ravaged by the elements, to food and tools that can be used to attract attention. In the following pages, you'll find the basic components of assembling that pack as well as tips to insure that you give yourself the maximum chance of survival in just about any situation.

Before you get overwhelmed, though, it's important to start today if you have nothing. Sort through what you have and start from there. A simple water proof Ziploc back with some gauze, alcohol, and band aids is a start. You can build from there once you've laid out a list of everything you should have.

Chapter 1 – Pack's

As the title of this book suggests, it's all about the kit and what you put inside it. If your kit is large enough, you can call it a pack. While you can spend a fair amount of money on advanced kits, a better strategy would be to either start from scratch or with a bare bone first aid kit and then supplement the kit with additional supplies.

For starters, you should have more than one kit. I recommend at least three, one for your home, one for your car or bike, and then one to take on your person in case you go hiking or will be an extended distance from your home or transportation. If you want just one kit, you should then pick a large pack for the home, which should have a smaller portable pack for your car, and yet an even smaller kit which you can remove to take on foot. Regardless of how you organize them, each of the smaller kits should still contain most of the same components just fewer of each item.

The thing about prepackaged kits or packs is that they are typically designed for specific circumstances. Some are more geared towards tending wounds, others are more focused on food and surviving the wild. To be fully prepared you'll need a bit of everything. As such, one strategy would be to buy three different basic kits for three different scenarios, and then borrow from each. You can then supplement each of the three with additional supplies. If you are starting from scratch, you will simply add more supplies of each item in your larger kits.

For packs stored on your person and in your car or bike, you want to make sure they are made of light and durable materials. Waterproof and sun proof material is also highly recommended. Larger packs stored in your home can be heavier and don't necessarily need to be sun proof, but they should be waterproof in the event of a flood.

Your packs should also include a checklist, preferably on the outside, but if not, you should have a checklist easily accessible on a secured pocket or lining on the inside, and your supplies should be dated. Dating your supplies is essential so you can prevent expired medicine or food. Even tools should be dated and periodically replaced from time to time.

Once your packs are fully stocked with supplies, which we'll discuss more in detail in further chapters, you should check your pack at a minimum of four times per year or once per quarter. This is to make sure you have all the supplies you need and that your supplies are still good and useful, but regardless of where you are with money or supplies, the main thing is to get started even if that means starting with just a waterproof zip lock bag with a few essentials.

Chapter 2 – Tools

For starters, I highly recommend a Swiss army knife. A basic pocket knife may work for your personal kit, but the one in your car or bike should have a multi-functional knife for multiple purposes. This is like having your own utility belt in a much smaller space. It will be invaluable for many unforeseen circumstances. A manual food can opener should also be included if your Swiss army or pocket knife doesn't contain that feature.

Make sure that your knife is legal in your jurisdiction. When using the actual blade, always cut away from yourself and others. Knives can be used not only as a weapon but also for things such as cutting ropes and bandages, opening things, making a fire (bow drill), cutting branches and tarp for shelters, and numerous other things.

You should also have a compass or other tool for navigation. Smart phones with GPS apps will do you no good if cell towers are down. A basic compass and a physical map of your area plus a national map are needed.

You should also include a method to contact someone in case of an emergency. Again, if you cell phone is not working for whatever reason, signal flares will be essential. For smaller kits, a reflecting mirror and a whistle can work as well. I recommend all three. Also add glow sticks for visibility in the dark.

Your pack at home or in your car should include WD-40. Your personal pack should include some type of non-oil based lubricant. This is extremely helpful if you find yourself stuck or you have a mechanical device that is stuck and immobile.

In addition, you should have fish hooks and a sewing kit. You will have numerous uses for these besides fishing or sewing. They can be used for medical purposes as well as retrieving items.

A solar powered battery recharger is important for your two larger kits. You should also have solar powered or hand powered flashlights and radios. A disposable cell phone or solar powered recharger with an adapter for your cell phone is also recommended. There are various methods of making your own if you are unable to find one that is ready made. Just be sure that you check to make sure that it works before you add it to your kit.

Duct tape is another must. This tool has a seemingly infinite number of uses. Don't leave home without it. Just make sure that your tape, like everything else, has been dated. It won't do you any good if it's no longer sticky.

Hollow tubing is also helpful. I would include different sizes, both narrow and wide. Narrow tubing can be used to open up airways in cases of blockages from food. It can also be used to create makeshift intravenous bags to deliver food, water and medicine.

Wider tubing can be used to transport gas, oil, water, and other liquids. It can be used as a makeshift underwater breathing apparatus or to ventilate an area or siphon air through a small space.

A rescue tool is also useful, especially in cars. These can be used to cut seat belts and break glass in the event of an accident or submersion under water. In cars, a jack and spare tire are also necessary. Those along with jumper cables should be in every car.

I would also include a basic tool kit. You can find small multifunctional kits that contain things like hammers and screwdrivers. You should also make sure you have nails and screws as well. A nail gun and stapler are also handy, both of which have medical and protective applications. Include a plunger, and insect bait. You'll be surprised at the applications of both.

Finally, you should have a survival manual. It may sound silly, but it could save your life. Have one for your home and car, and a mini packet for your personal kit. It's a great idea to actually read the guides prior to adding them, but no one has a perfect memory, so find a good guide and bring it with you. If you're out of cell range and you need it, you'll thank yourself that you did when the time comes.

Chapter 3 – Medicine

You can't have a survival medical kit without medicine and first aid, so here we go. I will only briefly reference items mentioned in other section for medical uses, starting with duct tape.

Duct tape can be used to close a wound, among other things. To go with the duct tape, you should have something that you can use to suture the wound first, namely, butterfly sutures. If you have a large cut or gash, this is a great way to close the wound temporarily until you can reach a hospital to see if you need real stitches. For smaller cuts, this may be all you need to close the wound. Just make sure that you clean the wound first with water and alcohol or disinfectants.

You should also have absorbent compress dressings, at least two for each kit. Too much moisture can lead to infection, so after the wounded is cleaned and disinfected, make sure you absorb any excess moisture, which can also weaken adhesive seals from bandages.

Make sure you have plenty of bandages. At least 25 in various sizes and shapes are recommended by the Red Cross. I would include at least twice that many so you have separate them for your portable kits. You should also include two three inches and two four-inch roller bandages for larger wounds.

That brings us to a very important section, which is disinfectants and infection preventions. Soap and water is the minimum you need to clean a wound, and this should be included in your kit, but you should also have either alcohol or peroxide. Antiseptic wipes are an excellent option, especially for smaller kits. Still, I would include alcohol in at least your home kit. I also recommend antiseptic creams, which you can apply periodically and can speed up healing.

You should also have something to cover the wound such as gauze. Smaller band aids are also useful, but medical gauze is more effective for the larger wounds. You should also include quick clotting gauze. This will aid in clotting for cuts and gashes. Other sections also mentioned coverings, such as bandanas, which can be used in a pinch if you are out of gauze or missing it for some reason. Other coverings may work as well if you have no other option.

Other guides may recommend trying to get an advance prescription of antibiotics, but I recommend against this. This is the sort of thing that has created antibiotic resistant strains of bacteria, and you also do not have the medical expertise to decide if you need one or which type would be preferred. Stick with prevention on this count.

I would also recommend against any other prescription medication, with the exception of making sure you have an existing supply of any long term prescription drugs you may be taking. Stick with the over the counter medication. Keep it safe, and keep it legal.

Also, don't fall into the trap of natural or homeopathic medicine. That isn't real medication, and it won't help you one bit if you need something in an emergency. Natural medications are also not uniform in their ingredients, the amount of the ingredients, and can have interactions with other drugs. Stick with what is supported by evidence based science. That doesn't mean you can used herbs in the wild. If you are aware of specific drugs or substances contained in plants that are scientifically supported to improve or aid in healing, such as aloe vera, feel free to use them in you have access.

What you should have is lot of over the counter medication, which I'll discuss in a moment. You should also be aware of any allergies as well as common side effects or interactions between various drugs as well as any prescription drugs you may be taking. It may be a good idea to look up the medications ahead of time so you can select types that you know will not interact with any drugs you are taking now.

Along those lines, I would also include a medical manual for emergencies. Your survival manual, which you should have as well, will cover some basics, but I would add a specific one for medicine. Again, you may not feel the need to take a paper manual in lieu of a digital version, but you may not also have access to a fully charged phone or electronic device, so don't skimp on this one.

The first type of medication you should have is pain medication. As mentioned before, stick with the legal variety. Aleve, Aspirin, Tylenol, and Ibuprofen are a must. Aleve works great, but if something works better for you, feel free to include that as well.

For muscle pain, cold and heat pads work great. They've already been mentioned in other sections, so you should have them on hand. You can also include muscle cream for additional relief if that works better for you. I would also add skin creams, such as hydrocortisone as well as topical anesthetics, such as oral gel, for dental or oral relief. You should also include Calamine lotion for rashes. Don't forget to throw in insect repellant as well.

Another category of drugs you should include is antihistamines for allergies. You can add something like Benadryl, but I would also include something for severe allergic reactions such as an EpiPen for things like nut, shellfish, or bee allergies.

Burns are another category that you should be prepared for. I would include both sunscreen, but prevention of sunburns, as well as aloe vera gels for sun damage and general skin healing. You should also have medicated burn creams for more severe first and second degree burns.

In addition, make sure you include stomach and digestive medications such as anti-diarrhea medication, laxatives, antacids, anti-nausea, and anti-gas meds. Pepto-Bismol is a good all-around stomach medication, but include whatever you prefer.

Anti-cold medications should also be included. Add items such as decongestants as well as fever and cough suppressants. Nighttime and daytime options are a plus.

You should also be prepared for fractures and broken bones. In the tools and ropes section, you should have netting or ropes that can be used for setting and tying, but you should also include some inexpensive SAM splints which are often used by emergency medical personnel.

You should have a Swiss Army knife, or at least a pocket knife. Check to see if you have tweezers or nail clippers included in the knife. If not, stock them separately.

A few additional items include a stethoscope, scalpel, needles and syringe, ear or bulb syringe (for cleaning out the nose or earwax), thermometer, Q-tips, eyewash and dressing, safety pins, cotton balls, as well as grooming supplies.

One important thing to remember about the medical section of your kit is that your items should be dated. You may not need to write the date on the items themselves, but you should have an insert with each category dated so you can periodically replace expired and old items. Medicine does expire. It can lose its effectiveness and even break down chemically into other substances, with can create other side effects or interactions.

Also, make sure you have three sets of medical supplies, one for your larger home kit, as well as one for your car or bike and one for your person. That means at a minimum, you should have three of each item or three items for the same purpose, which you can separate into smaller sections as needed.

I would also recommend that you education yourself in first aid. Learn how to do basic CPR and the Heimlich maneuver. Read and review your first aid kit and medical manual so you are familiar with it and know where to find it quickly if you need to brush up on the specifics.

Finally, make sure you have copies of any relevant medical consent forms and something to write with. Hopefully you won't need to use this, but include them anyway just in case.

Chapter 4 – Ropes

Ropes can be used for a variety of things. They can be used in conjunction with a bandana as a tourniquet. They allow you to climb or descend obstacles for movement or escape. Ropes can hold you in place during a flood, prevent you from falling, or rescue others. They can hoist objects, be used for hunting, kindling, signaling, or numerous other purposes including medical applications such as setting a fracture.

Survival rope packs can be purchased for as little as five dollars. Be careful though, because different ropes do different things, so you need to educate yourself one which type of rope is best for certain situations such as strength, water resistance, weight, etc. I recommend more than one type of rope. A combination of two or three ropes is preferable.

Of all the ropes, you should include paracord (used in parachutes) as your primary rope. Include this no matter what. It is extremely lightweight, durable, strong, an versatile, which is the key in any survival event.

Paracord can serve the function of hiking, building traps, fishing, holding or securing gear, tying a tarp, sewing, trip wire, flossing, creating a pulley, sling, catapult, building a ladder or hammock, making a raft, be used as a bow drill for a fire, repairing broken equipment, making shelter, or making a stretcher.

Like many things, though, you get what you pay for. Make sure you invest in quality paracord. When the time comes, you'll be grateful that you did.

Good secondary ropes can include things like bungee cord, climbing ropes, or tow straps (not actually a rope, but should be included in your car nonetheless).

Make sure that at a minimum, you include paracord in your car and home kits, and include more than one type of rope if you can.

Chapter 5 – Coverage

There are several items that should be included for coverage. The first is trash bags. These can be used as ponchos, storage, or other purposes. If you have a bright colored bag, such as the orange versions used by the transportation department, that's even better.

Another coverage item that should be included is a light-weight foil space blanket. This will be used for warmth as well as sleeping or hiding.

A bandana is also a surprisingly useful survival tool. They can do more than just hold your hair in place. They can keep you warm, work as a placeholder, carry items, be used as tinder or kindling for a fire, soak up water or sweat, alert others to an emergency, filter water, make a waste bag, be used as a bandage, extend cords, clean, block the sun, be used as a mask, mark trails, hold pots, or even be used as a weapon.

I would also include a hat. While you can use a bandana to cover your head, a separate hat should be included as coverage from the sun, wind, and rain. You may need the bandana for something else. Sunglasses and face paint should also be include for camouflage and protection against the elements.

You should also add an extra change of clothes. This should be self-explanatory. Add a pair of gloves as well. Surgical gloves should be in your personal pack, but your larger packs should include larger gloves for warmth or manual tasks.

In addition, I would include a water proof mat, such as a yoga matt. This can be used as insulation or to block smoke. A fabric blanket or towel should also be included, which can be used for warmth, to soak up water, as a partition, or an additional filter. It can also be used as additional kindling.

Another set of items you should include are absorbent pads for children, female needs, and the elderly. Be well stocked on these in cased of a prolonged period without access to a store or residence.

Shelter is another consideration, especially if you are injured or in extreme cold, heat, wind, dust, or other harsh weather. You can make your own make shift shelter with the items already discussed here and in earlier sections. Your trash bags and paracord could be used as a basic tarp or tent. Just make sure that you do a bit of research beforehand so you know how you can efficiently set it up.

Chapter 6 – Fire

Start with a magnifying glass. You can heat up paper and dry materials by concentrating the suns energy without the need for matches. This will be invaluable if you run out of matches or your matches get wet.

Matches are still useful, so add them too. I also recommend a big shot butane torch for your larger packs. This will come in handy for protection and hunting when you run out of food. This also means stocking up on a bit of butane. Start with a lighter for your smaller packs, but then work up to the butane torch for your car and home packs.

In addition, you should have some tinder or materials that can be used to set fire. Don't assume you'll always have materials from your environment. Without something that can be burned, there is no fire. If your emergency kit in your home or car is well stocked, you should also have additional items which can be used as kindling, such as a fabric blanket or towel, bandana, or spare clothes.

Smoke from fire can also be used for different things such as signaling for help. In addition, smoke can paralyze certain insects and wild creatures, such as certain bees or wasps.

You should also be prepared to not just start a fire, but escape from one. This means, you can use those same fabrics used for kindling as face masks. They can also be used to absorb water and keep you and your area damp if needed.

Protective goggles or glasses can also be used to protect your used in the event you need to make or escape from a fire. A fire blanket and mini fire-extinguisher should also be included in your auto or home kit.

Chapter 7 – Food & Water

Water and food are essential to survival, and you should have them in all your kits, including your personal kit. You should also have a plan to get more food and purify water if your existing supplies run out.

Water is more important than food, but clean water is even more important. This means you need purification tablets. You can treat at much as 25 quarts with a single bottle of the iodine based variety.

Another option would be a small amount of unscented bleach. A couple drops can purify a liter of water. There is a problem with bleach, though, in that it degrades over time. A better chemical is calcium hypochlorite. A one-pound bag of the stuff can purify 10,000 gallons of water and is more effective at killing other types of pathogens. The process is more involved, and I would only recommend it for your larger household kit. UV lighting devices, such as UVSteripen, can also disinfect water and cost as little as $40.

A portable filter is also useful if you can't use the above methods. You can find simple techniques to use coffee filters, crushed charcoal, small sand or pebbles, and then larger gravel in a water bottle or other container to quickly filter water in a rush.

The fall back, however, is always boiling water. If you have a way to heat up water with fire, such as matches or a magnifying glass, boil your water to kill bacteria, parasites, and other pathogens. Boiling water is the single most effective way to purify water. It won't, however, get rid of salt or heavy metals unless you use condensation capture methods after boiling. If you think your water may have lead, mercury, or other contaminants, I recommend using a filter prior to boiling, or desalinate your water by capturing condensation if you are getting water from the sea.

An emergency supply of food should be included in every kit. Start with the basics, freeze dried food packets with something that can make fire. Fire was already discussed in an earlier section of the book, but it will be very important if you find yourself in a situation where you are forced to find food beyond your existing supplies. Thoroughly cooking wild game will insure that you won't contract most diseases and infections.

Still, there are other options for food. A few protein or energy bars is a good start for a mini pack on the go, at least in the beginning. You can also find a 30 day supply of vitamin and mineral supplements for the food storage for as little as $30. This won't contain and the protein and sugars you'll need, but will give you the minimum necessary to keep going once your supply stock has run out. Hopefully by that time, you will have been rescued. If not, it will give you plenty of time and find or hunt for more food in the interim.

You should also add cold and heat packets. You can find light, cheap chemical packets which can be used not only for heating or cooling food and water, but they can also be used as cold and hot compresses for medical purposes.

A final discussion on food should also include what to do in the event that you find yourself with no supplies. In that instance, you want will need to find or hunt for food. The first rule of eating in the wild is not to eat something unless you are absolutely sure you know what it is. If you know the area, and are certain what you are eating is blackberries as opposed to poison berries of some variety you'll have an advantage. If you are unsure, follow the recommendations in the next paragraph.

If you are near a body of water, fishing can also be a life saver. Netting and capture methods may be more effective in the long term, but if you've stock the fish hook and thread, as recommended in earlier chapters, you'll have what you need to catch fish.

Skimming, filtering, and drying kelp or seaweed is an excellent way to supplement your food supply. They are high in many nutrients and will go a long way in providing you a long term food source if you need it.

If you must survive away from a body of water, eating higher on the food chain may save your life, but stick to small game. Small game requires less energy and is far safer than running around like a maniac trying to trap or spear wild bears deer.

If there are no plants that you know are edible, insects are never in short supply. Insects will supply you with the protein you need to keep going, and if you're well stocked on a 30-day supplement of vitamins and minerals you'll be in decent shape. Also, if you've stocked the recommended items in prior sections, you'll have all that you need to acquire insects and small game such as rabbits, raccoons, or squirrels. Usually, though, all you need to capture insects is a stick or a little bit of elbow grease.

Unless you are an expert on fruits and berries, I would skip the berries and go straight to finding nuts. Tree nuts provide an excellent source of fats and protein. To list a few, there are acorns, beechnuts, chestnuts, black walnuts, butternuts, and hickory nuts to name a few. The flavor can vary from tree to tree, and I recommend roasting them. Still, tree nuts can harbor hidden dangers. There are a few toxic nuts, such as the nut from the buckeye tree. One might also have allergic reactions to certain nuts, so make sure you know your allergies, and inform yourself on the nuts in your area.

Finally, I would include some type of container. Something like a hydro flask would work great, but you might want to include a bowl, utensils, and power towels as well.

Conclusion

Regardless of the situation, planning is always essential. The most basic planning is what you need to do before you are in a situation where you or a loved one are in an emergency. Whether it's preparation for a natural disaster, or something else, plan ahead by taking a few short steps to stock a basic medicine kit. That, along with the knowledge of first aid might save your life in many situations.

Make sure that your emergency kit includes smaller portable sub kits that can be used in your car and on your person. Educate yourself on how to use the items you have, and check often to make sure that your perishables are still good. While this may not save you in every instance, it will maximize your chances to survive as much as possible, which is all you can hope for.

As with most situations, a little preparation goes a long way. More importantly, the best advice I can give is to remain calm and conserve energy wherever possible. This will help prevent you from doing silly things and making stupid mistakes in the event of an emergency. It will also extend the time you need to survive or get rescued. Having a well-stocked emergency kit can only assist in that endeavor, so long as you know where it is at all times and that your kit is out of the reach of children.

OR Go to this URL

http://zbit.ly/1WBb1Ek